NursetoNurse 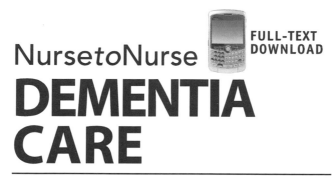 **FULL-TEXT DOWNLOAD**

DEMENTIA CARE

FOLLOW THESE INSTRUCTIONS TO DOWNLOAD:

1) Use your Web browser to go to:
http://www.mhnursetonurse.com

2) Register now

3) Fill in the required fields

4) Enter your unique registration code below

5) Download the software and sync into your handheld device

Code Listed Here

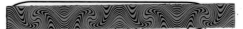

NOTE: BOOK IS NOT RETURNABLE ONCE SCRATCH-OFF IS REMOVED

Scratch off coating above to reveal your unique code to download your mobile device software.

See above for complete directions.

If you have any problems accessing your download, please email: techsolutions@mhedu.com

P/N 9780071590822
007159082X
part of set
ISBN 978-0-07-148432-9
MHID 0-07-148432-9

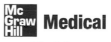

mcgraw-hillmedical.com

Nurse to Nurse
DEMENTIA CARE

Nurse to Nurse
DEMENTIA CARE

Cynthia D. Steele, MPH, RN

Assistant Professor, Department of Psychiatry and Behavioral Sciences,
The Johns Hopkins University Schools of Medicine and Nursing

Senior Faculty, The Copper Ridge Institute
Baltimore, Maryland

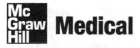
Medical

New York Chicago San Francisco Lisbon London Madrid Mexico City
Milan New Delhi San Juan Seoul Singapore Sydney Toronto

Nurse to Nurse: Dementia Care

1 2 3 4 5 6 7 8 9 0   DOC/DOC   12 11 10 9

Set ISBN: 978-0-07-148432-9; MHID: 0-07-148432-9
Book ISBN: 978-0-07-159081-5; MHID: 0-07-159081-1
Card ISBN: 978-0-07-159082-2; MHID: 0-07-159082-X

This book was set in Berkeley Book by Glyph International.
The editors were Joseph Morita and Karen G. Edmonson.
The production supervisor was Catherine H. Saggese.
Project management was provided by Ekta Dixit, Glyph International.
The book designer was Eve Siegel.
The cover designer was David Dell'Accio.
The indexer was Robert Swanson.
RR Donnelley was printer and binder.

This book is printed on acid-free paper.

Library of Congress Cataloging-in-Publication Data

Steele, Cynthia, 1947-
    Nurse to nurse. Dementia care / Cynthia D. Steele.
        p. ; cm.
    Includes bibliographical references and index.
    ISBN-13: 978-0-07-148432-9 (pbk.)
    ISBN-10: 0-07-148432-9
    1. Dementia—Nursing.   2. Dementia—Patients—Care.   I. Title. II.
Title: Dementia care.
    [DNLM: 1. Dementia—nursing.   WM 220 S814n 2010]
    RC521.S74 2010
    616.8'30231—dc22

                                                    2009046501

McGraw-Hill books are available at special quantity discounts to use as premiums and sales promotions, or for use in corporate training programs. To contact a representative please visit the Contact Us pages at http://www.mhprofessional.com.

Contents

Preface

After my over 25 years of experience in the care of those with dementia and their families, it is apparent that an easy reference book is needed for those who provide direct care. The need for informed care is significant as those affected can live as long as 20 years until death. Many of these years are spent in a very debilitated state. As the science moves forward in an attempt to understand the underlying pathologic mechanism of dementing disorders, day-to-day care must be provided. Persons with dementia will be encountered by nurses across health care settings.

My philosophy is that even those who are severely debilitated deserve informed and respectful care until the end of their lives. That care includes special skills not only from medical/surgical perspectives but also neurological and psychiatric expertise. An underlying tenet is that effective care is "person centered." It is to understand the person's life before the illness; their interests and prior experiences will allow one to provide the most effective care.

This quick reference guide is meant to be of practical use by front line workers to solve day-to-day care problems. Each chapter begins with key points and further detailed discussions of each.

The book begins with an overview of the clinical characteristics of the many diseases causing dementia, how they can be recognized, and care tailored to them. An especially important chapter of this book informs caregivers on how to understand behavior problems and how to devise care that minimizes or prevents them.

Another valuable component of this book is the series of Family Guidelines. In my experience, both professional and family caregivers are often overloaded by complicated care directions. The Guidelines in this book are meant to be reprinted and made available as appropriate to clinical and family caregivers to focus on one area of care at a time. They can be used as an educational tool for staff and also given to families as they continue day-to-day care after discharge from a health care facility.

In the past, the determination of a case of dementia led to the search for a medication that could stop it or slow the progress of the disease. Currently, diagnostic procedures have been formulated and are quite accurate during life. Unfortunately, the medications to treat the underlying dementia have not proven successful in either significantly slowing the progression of the illness or stopping it. Scientists are now focused on ways to prevent the disease from starting or methods to delay the onset. To date those efforts have not been fruitful.

So, the day-to-day care of the millions of persons affected by dementia continues and is carried out by nurses, aides, companions and family members. This is difficult and challenging work. While we await a cure or prevention, the goal of care is to provide positive moments for patients, activity that is stimulating and meticulous nursing care all given with knowledge and respect for the life the person lived prior to becoming ill.

It is my hope that this book will provide clear direction to caregivers and improve the lives of the millions of persons affected by dementia.

Cynthia D. Steele, MPH, RN

Chapter 1
DEMENTIA BASICS

Cynthia D. Steele

Key Points

- Impact of dementia on health care
- Normal brain function versus brain function in dementia
- The meaning of dementia
- Causes of dementia

UNDERSTANDING DEMENTIA

The population of the United States and other countries is aging rapidly. Accompanying this aging population is a dramatic rise in the number of cases of dementia. *Dementia* is a general term for a disorder characterized by global intellectual deterioration. Because of the rapid aging of the population, the number of people with dementia is expected to increase dramatically in the next 10 to 20 years. In fact, dementia is now the most common mental disorder in the elderly.

Dementia by the Numbers

- More than 5 million people in the United States have dementia.
- At the age of 65, approximately 7% of elderly experience dementia.
- Between ages 75 and 85, the number doubles to about 16% of elderly.

- Over the age of 85, at least half of the population has dementia.
- More than 27.7 million people worldwide have dementia.[1]

In the years to come, a large percentage of patients will be elderly (older than age 65) and at high risk of having dementia. This is true across all practice settings and nursing specialties. Nurses who specialize in specific disorders will care for many older patients likely to suffer from dementia, as shown in the percentages of elderly patients in specialty care:[2]

- Oncology   63%
- Cardiology   60%
- Urology   53%
- Ophthalmology   52%[2]

The aging population makes up the majority of patients in a variety of health care settings. The percentage of elderly patients in different health care settings is listed here.[2]

- Ambulatory care   65%
- Hospitals   48%
- ICUs   46%
- Home care   80%
- Nursing homes   90%
- Assisted living   70%

Impact on Health Care System

Dementia also has a major impact on the health care system as a whole.[2] When compared with normal elderly, older adults with dementia have:

- 3 times more hospital admissions
- 21.8 times higher hospital costs
- 3.1 times higher home health costs
- 2 to 3 times the length of hospital stay

Dementia is a common disorder with major ramifications for nurses, who will need the special knowledge and skills to care for such patients across the health care system.

NORMAL AGING, THINKING, AND MEMORY

It is vital for nurses to understand how the normal brain works, as the impairments that are common in dementia are related to the location of damage in the brain.

As a review, the brain has two hemispheres, right and left. Figure 1-1 shows the left hemisphere, with the front of the brain at the left and the back at the right. Table 1-1 reviews the normal functions of each part of the brain shown in Figure 1-1. This information can alert you to which parts of the brain are damaged in your patients with dementia.

WHAT IS DEMENTIA?

Forgetfulness and disorientation were once considered a normal part of aging. It was believed that if one lived long enough, such impairments were inevitable. Currently, dementia is considered an abnormal state with many causes that can often be identified. A well-accepted definition of dementia is:

> A global intellectual decline of sufficient severity to impair social and or occupational functioning that occurs in normal consciousness.[3]

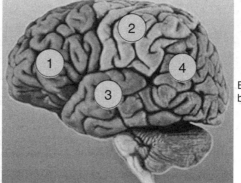

Figure 1-1   Lobes of the brain.

Table 1-1   Functions in a Normal Brain Versus a Diseased Brain

Part of the Brain	Normal Functions	Impact in Disease States	Impact on Behavior
1. Frontal lobe	• Organizing tasks • Regulation of manners • Inhibition of impulses • Decision-making	• Inability to sequence task • Inability to regulate and inhibit behavior	• Putting underwear over clothing • Eating from another's plate • Cussing, swearing
2. Parietal lobe	• Sensory perception • Movement	• Inability to interpret tactile sensations • Difficulty in performing learned motor movements	• Inability to identify spoiled food by smell • Inability to sense one's skin is being burned • Difficulty in orienting body to get into a car
3. Temporal lobe	• Memory • Rage	• Inability to form new memories • Emotional response	• Asking questions over and over • Sudden reactions to minor events with episodes of rage
4. Occipital lobe	• Recognizing what you see	• Inability to recognize objects, places, people	• May not recognize spouse; may be afraid of him or her • Constantly wants to go home • Unable to recognize what is and is not food

There are four key elements to the definition of dementia:

1. **Global impairment.** The impairments in dementia are global. Impairments occur in more than just memory. Most dementia patients experience impairments in reasoning, using and understanding language, recognizing what one perceives through the senses, coordinating learned motor movements, planning, and decision-making.

2. **Decline.** The impairments represent a decline from a previous level of functioning. To recognize decline, it is crucial for the nurse to know the patient's previous level of functioning. Methods of assessment for determining decline are presented in Chapter 3. Patients who are mentally retarded are not necessarily demented as they age. The exception to this are people with Down syndrome, all of whom will have the pathology of Alzheimer disease in their brains at 40 years and older.

3. **Severity.** Impairments are severe enough to interfere with normal functioning in everyday life. Examples are a person who was living independently and begins to make poor financial decisions or forgets how to cook a meal, although the person could previously perform those tasks. Getting lost while driving can also indicate severe impairment.

4. **Normal consciousness.** These impairments occur in a normal state of consciousness; patients are awake and alert. This is distinguished from an abnormal state of consciousness, such as drowsiness, stupor, or coma, seen in delirium. Delirious patients wax and wane in their consciousness and ability to pay attention to the world around them. A common example is a postsurgery patient who must be aroused to take a medication but quickly falls asleep as a result of anesthesia and pain medicine.

CAUSES OF DEMENTIA

There are many brain disorders that cause dementia. The currently recognized causes of dementia are represented in the pie chart shown in Figure 1-2. Each type has a distinctive profile of symptoms and course.

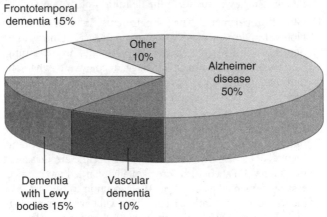

Figure 1-2   Causes of dementia by percentage of patients.

Alzheimer Disease

Alzheimer disease (AD) is the most common cause of dementia and thus the most common type that nurses encounter in clinical practice. AD is an incurable neurodegenerative disease. The hallmark pathology of AD includes amyloid plaques and neurofibrillary tangles in the brain. One also sees general shrinkage of the brain and a decrease in the number of functioning neurons.

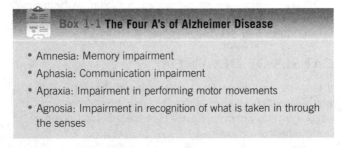

Box 1-1 The Four A's of Alzheimer Disease

- Amnesia: Memory impairment
- Aphasia: Communication impairment
- Apraxia: Impairment in performing motor movements
- Agnosia: Impairment in recognition of what is taken in through the senses

Table 1-2   Stages of Alzheimer Disease

Stage 1	Stage 2	Stage 3
Amnesia: Short-term memory loss	• *Aphasia:* Impaired communication both in producing language and in understanding language. Vague, empty speech • *Apraxia:* Impairment performing learned motor movements such as putting a key in a lock and buttoning clothing • *Agnosia:* Difficulty recognizing the world around them. Inability to recognize familiar people such as relatives	• Short-term and long-term memory loss • Ability to say only a few words • Inability to perform self-care • Difficulty chewing and swallowing • Difficulty walking

Currently, there is no cure for Alzheimer disease, and treatments that are available may impact the symptoms but do not slow down the disease process. Alzheimer disease affects different patients in different ways, and progresses steadily until patients are completely disabled. The disease typically progresses through three stages (Table 1-2).

Patients with AD live 4 to 20 years after diagnosis. The most common causes of death are from aspiration of food or fluids into the lungs and from the complications of immobility, as patients are unable to walk.

Vascular Dementia

Vascular dementia (VD), resulting from impaired blood supply to the brain, is the second most common form of dementia. The most common cause of VD is a series of small, often undetectable strokes in the brain. Such strokes disrupt the flow of blood, oxygen, and nutrients to the affected area. The clinical picture of dementia emerges when a total of 50 mL of brain tissue is damaged. VD can occur along with AD, and is then called *mixed dementia*. The changes in functioning can occur suddenly or gradually as more and more tissue is damaged.

Symptoms

The symptoms of VD vary according to the area of the brain damaged by the disruption of blood flow, nutrients, and oxygen. The symptoms that point to vascular disease being the cause of dementia are:

- Abrupt onset of symptoms, often following a stroke
- Stepwise course with periods of stability, often called *plateaus*
- Dizziness
- Focal neurologic signs, such as weakness of an arm or leg
- Early gait disturbance
- Emotional lability (mood swings)
- Difficulty in making decisions
- Fluctuations in functioning, often called good and bad days
- Patchy impairments, such as language more impaired than memory
- Increased likelihood of developing depression
- Self-awareness of mental and physical problems late into the illness
- Arterial disease elsewhere in the body, such as in the coronary arteries

Prognosis

There is no current way to restore the function of the brain in areas damaged by the strokes of VD, and there is some evidence that having VD increases a patient's later risk of developing AD. Further damage can be prevented by addressing the risk factors for stroke. These include managing diabetes and hypertension, losing weight, exercising, avoiding smoking, and controlling heart disease and high cholesterol.

The course of VD is difficult to predict. Death usually occurs due to a vascular event such as a large stroke or myocardial infarction. Patients with VD live about 8 to 15 years. Even though the cause of VD is different from AD, patients eventually have a progressive decline until death.

Lewy Body Dementia

Lewy body dementia (LBD) is characterized by progressive cognitive decline. Other features distinct to those with LBD are:

- Fluctuations in consciousness
- Recurrent visual hallucinations
- Parkinsonism motor symptoms[4]

The fluctuations in consciousness are evidenced by periods of drowsiness, lethargy, and staring into space. Nurses are often concerned that the staring into space is an early sign of aggression. This is typically not a deliberate behavior to threaten the nurse, but a result of the brain disease. Patients with LBD often prefer to spend long periods of time in bed sleeping. The visual hallucinations are often quite vivid, and patients can describe them in detail. In many cases, the hallucinations are not frightening or disturbing. Patients with LBD are very sensitive to neuroleptic medications, and thus hallucinations are difficult to treat.

The parkinsonism motor symptoms result in slowed movement and poor balance, resulting in falls and muscle rigidity. In some cases these symptoms are helped by the use of the same medications used for Parkinson disease such as levodopa. These symptoms progress as the disease worsens.

Lewy body dementia is described as having three stages: early, middle, and late.

- **Early stage:** Forgetfulness, poor concentration, unstable gait and depression.
- **Middle stage:** Worsening cognition that fluctuates and is often worse at night. Visual and auditory hallucinations and paranoid delusions. Falls become more frequent.
- **Late stage:** Rapid progression of cognitive decline, increase in frequency of behavioral disturbance, shouting, and aggression. Death occurs within months, in many cases, and is most often secondary to aspiration pneumonia.

Treatment of LBD focuses on the Parkinson-like features and the hallucinations and paranoid delusions. Medications approved for Alzheimer disease are often used and are helpful for cognitive dysfunction in some patients.

Frontotemporal Dementia

Frontotemporal dementia (FTD) primarily affects the frontal and anterior temporal lobes. In contrast to other types of dementia, personality, behavior, and language ability are affected first, and memory is often normal until late into the disease. As a result, the following features are characteristic of FTD:

- Disinhibited and inappropriate social behavior
- Inappropriate sexual behavior
- Loss of concern about personal hygiene and appearance
- Major increase in appetite and weight gain
- Apathy
- Lack of concern for others
- Compulsive and repetitive behaviors such as touching, collecting things
- Putting objects into mouth
- Memory loss (this evolves after the above symptoms)

Other Causes of Dementia

Around 10% of dementia cases are caused by more rare conditions described in Table 1-3.

CONDITIONS THAT MIMIC DEMENTIA

There are several common conditions that mimic dementia but may be treatable and reversible. In the process of a diagnostic workup, such conditions are ruled out by exams, lab work, and brain imaging before the diagnosis of Alzheimer disease is made. These conditions include:

Table 1-3   Other Causes of Dementia and Key Clinical Features

Cause	Clinical Features
Multiple sclerosis (MS)	• Impairments in information processing, memory retrieval, decision-making, and planning • Poor regulation of mood • 16%–20% of MS patients have mood disorders, particularly major depression • Delusions and hallucinations are rare • Lack of concern about impairment
Parkinson disease	• Decrease in processing and mental flexibility—that is, persons are slow to respond • Apathy and social withdrawal • Impairments in verbal output • 30%–60% develop depression • 30% have visual hallucinations of groups of people or animals • Delusions can occur as a result of treatment with anti-Parkinson medications
Creutzfeldt–Jakob disease (CJD)	• Personality change and disinhibition occur first • Rapid decline • Myoclonus (involuntary jerking of muscles and limbs) • Death within months to 6 years
Huntington disease	• Inherited neurologic degenerative disorder • Dance-like movements, involuntary movements • Poor coordination • Frequent falls • Apathy • Slowness of thinking • Recall impaired • High rates of depression and mania

(Continued)

Table 1-3   Other Causes of Dementia and Key Clinical Features
(*Continued*)

Cause	Clinical Features
Normal-pressure hydrocephalus (NPH)	• Dementia • Gait disturbance • Difficulty walking, broad-based magnetic gait • Urinary incontinence • Onset early 70s • Enlarged ventricles identified on brain imaging • Treatment is placement of shunt in brain to decrease pressure
Human immuno-deficiency virus (HIV)	• Memory loss • Slowed mental processing • Difficulty with planning • Apathy, social withdrawal • Cognitive impairment occurs much more often if CD4 count below 400

- Delirium, often a reaction to medications or dehydration
- Thyroid disease—hyperthyroidism or hypothyroidism
- Infections, such as urinary tract infection
- Anemia
- Vitamin B_{12} deficiency
- Depression
- Brain tumors
- Vasculitis

DIAGNOSIS OF DEMENTIA

The standard approach to establishing a diagnosis of dementia includes the following:

- History of the present illness
- Direct cognitive testing to establish decline

- Psychiatric evaluation to rule out depression and other mental disorders
- Neurologic evaluation to rule out strokes, Parkinson disease, and other neurologic conditions
- Laboratory tests to detect metabolic abnormalities such as thyroid disease
- Brain imaging to detect tumors
- Medical evaluation, including careful review of prescription and over-the-counter medications and herbs

Many patients in long-term care will have a diagnosis of dementia without an evaluation, and the specific cause of the dementia may not be known.

REFERENCES

1. Gallo JJ, Liebowitz BD. The epidemiology of common late-life mental disorders in the community: Themes for the new century. *Psychiatric Services*.1999;50(9):1158-1166.
2. Kuehn BM. Effort underway to prepare physicians to care for growing elderly population. *JAMA*. 2009;302(7):727-728.
3. Rabins PV, Lyketsos CG, Steele CD. *Practical dementia care*. New York: Oxford University Press; 2006.
4. National Institute of Neurological and Communication Disorders and Stroke, Rabins PV, Lyketsos CG, Steele CD. *Practical Dementia Care*. New York: Oxford University Press; 1999.

Chapter 2

COMMON COMPLICATIONS of DEMENTIA

Cynthia D. Steele

Key Points

- Significance of complications
- Finding the cause of complications
- Providing ideal care for patients with complications of dementia

Patients with dementia experience difficulties in memory, reasoning, planning, and caring for themselves. In addition, the majority of patients will experience one or more common complications of dementia, described in Tables 2-1 and 2-2.

The course of dementia with complications involves a sudden change in the patient's ability to think, remember, and function. These complications of dementia are often more troublesome to patients and families than the dementia alone. They

Table 2-1   Prevalence of Dementia Complications

Complication	Prevalence (%)
Delirium	22–89[1]
Depression	40[2]
Hallucinations and delusions	20–50[3]
Mania	2[4]
Apathy	15[5]

Table 2-2 Features of Common Complications of Dementia

Type	When	Onset	Duration	Defining Features	Clinical Features
Delirium	Anytime	Sudden	Hours/days	Abnormal fluctuating level of consciousness	Drowsiness, stupor, coma
Depression	Early	Gradual	Weeks/months	Sustained low mood, irritability	Withdrawal, tearfulness
Hallucinations	Middle	Sudden	Days to weeks	Seeing things, hearing voices	Looking at wall and screaming, attempting to leave the room
Delusions	Middle/late	Sudden	Days to weeks	False fixed beliefs	Suspicious ideas
Illusions	Middle/late	Sudden	Briefly	Misperceptions of stimuli in the environment	Looking at a robe draped over a chair, "get that man out of my room"
Mania	Early/middle	Gradual	Days to weeks	Increased level of mood	Irritability, rapid pacing, less need for sleep
Apathy	Middle/late	Gradual	Days to weeks	Patients won't get out of bed in morning	Will not partake in previously enjoyed activities

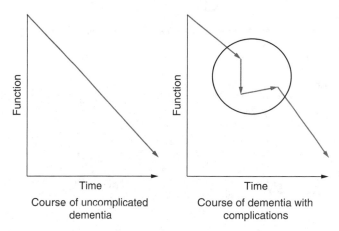

Figure 2-1   Course of uncomplicated and complicated dementia.

are often the reason patients are taken to the ED, seen in physicians' offices, evaluated by home care nurses, and admitted to hospitals (see Figure 2-1).

DELIRIUM

Delirium Defined

Patients who have dementia alone, have normal consciousness. In contrast, the hallmark of delirium is a state of abnormal consciousness. This is fluctuating and may include hypervigilant, drowsy, stuporous, and comatose states of consciousness, as shown in Figure 2-2. Specifically, delirium is an acute confusional state with an abnormal level of consciousness indicated by:

• Sudden change in cognitive function
• Waxing and waning of attentiveness
• Frequently abnormal sleep/wake cycles (awake during night, sleeping all day)
• Evidence of relationship to medical condition

Hypervigilant ——► Awake ——► Drowsy ——► Stupor ——► Coma

- Hypervigilant: The patient who is easily startled and stays up all night
- Awake: Awake and alert during day, asleep at night. This is a stable state.
- Drowsy: Sleepy most of the time but can be easily awakened
- Stupor: Asleep all the time and difficult to arouse
- Coma: Deep unconsciousness, unable to arouse

Figure 2-2   Consciousness continuum.

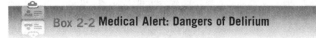

Box 2-1 Comparing Delirium and Dementia

The key difference between delirium and dementia is that in delirium, the patient has an abnormal and fluctuating level of consciousness. In dementia, patients are awake and alert and their level of consciousness is stable.

A demented patient with delirium may be difficult to arouse from sleep and may rapidly fall asleep again. The patient who stays awake all night and day and is easily startled is also experiencing an abnormal level of consciousness. Features of delirium and dementia are listed in Table 2-3.

Box 2-2 Medical Alert: Dangers of Delirium

Delirium is a serious and potentially life-threatening syndrome that must be attended to promptly. If it is ignored and assumed to be "just more dementia," the course of the underlying medical condition will worsen to potentially fatal consequences.

Table 2-3   Features of Delirium Versus Dementia

Feature	Delirium	Dementia
Onset	Sudden	Gradual
Duration	Hours/days	Months/years
Attention	Impaired	Normal
Consciousness	Fluctuating	Clear and stable
Speech	Incoherent	Ordered but may not make sense

Features of Delirium

- Abnormal and fluctuating level of consciousness
- Inattentiveness
- Distractibility
- Increased confusion and disorientation
- Lethargy or hyperactivity
- Rapid fluctuations of mood
- Visual hallucinations

Common Causes of Delirium

- Infections: Skin, respiratory, dental, renal
- Metabolic abnormalities: Hyperglycemia, hypoglycemia, electrolyte abnormalities
- Dehydration
- Medication side effects and interactions, most commonly from the following:
  — Antipsychotic medications
  — Anti-anxiety medications
  — Pain medications, narcotics
  — Anticholinergic medications
  — Anesthesia

Care of Patients with Delirium

DOs	DON'Ts
• Identify the cause and treat it. See Figure 2-3 for a suggested approach.	• Assume the change in consciousness is normal.
	• Ignore the change in consciousness.
	• Fail to inform the nurse or doctor.

Box 2-3 How to Conduct a Body Audit

1. Undress and visually inspect the patient.

2. Gently touch and inspect all body systems and observe for guarding of any body part. Look for rashes and bruises.

3. Listen to bowel sounds, listen to lungs, palpate bladder, and inspect the color and odor of urine to identify possible infections. Observe whether the color or odor of the urine has changed.

4. Carefully inspect the mouth to identify gum infections, decaying teeth, and sores.

5. If the patient is mobile, watch the patient walk to identify possible fractures that are unreported.

Significance of Delirium

• Demented patients are at high risk.

• Delirium is often not recognized promptly especially if patient is lethargic and quiet.

• Change in mental status and level of consciousness is often the FIRST SIGN OF A SERIOUS MEDICAL CONDITION.

- Risk of mortality is high.
- Unsafe behaviors are common, such as attempts to flee frightening hallucinations.

Delirium: Myths, and Reality in the Hospital?[1]

MYTH: "Older people get confused in the hospital."
REALITY: Delirium may be the sole indicator of serious illness.

MYTH: "Oriented times one, must be Alzheimer."
REALITY: Baseline functioning rarely known by clinical staff.

MYTH: "Hallmarks of delirium are agitation, hallucinations, and inappropriate behavior."
REALITY: More often, patients are lethargic.

MYTH: "Patient was confused last night but now seems with it, so nothing is wrong."
REALITY: A key feature of delirium is fluctuating course![6]

DEPRESSION

Depression Defined

Another common and serious complication of dementia is depression. Many think this is a reasonable reaction to realizing that one has dementia or a reaction to moving to a nursing home. This is unlikely the case, because of the diffuse brain damage suffered by patients with dementia.

Common Features of Depression in Dementia

- Low mood
- Irritability
- Non-sad; patient won't complain of feeling sad

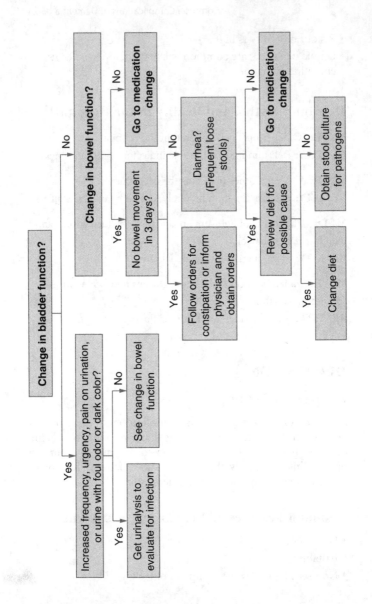

Change in bladder function?

Yes → Increased frequency, urgency, pain on urination, or urine with foul odor or dark color?

Yes → Get urinalysis to evaluate for infection

No → See change in bowel function

No → **Change in bowel function?**

No → **Go to medication change**

Yes → No bowel movement in 3 days?

Yes → Follow orders for constipation or inform physician and obtain orders

No → Diarrhea? (Frequent loose stools)

No → **Go to medication change**

Yes → Review diet for possible cause

Yes → Change diet

No → Obtain stool culture for pathogens

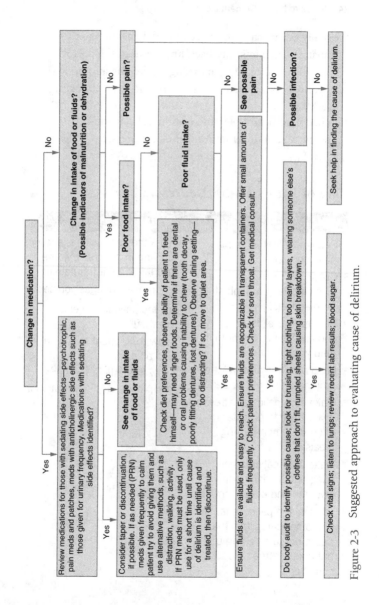

Change in medication?

Yes → Review medications for those with sedating side effects—psychotrophic, pain meds and patches, meds with anticholinergic side effects such as those given for urinary frequency. Medications with sedating side effects identified?

Yes → Consider taper or discontinuation, if possible. If as needed (PRN) meds given frequently to calm patient try to avoid giving them and use alternative methods, such as distraction, walking, activity. If PRN meds must be used, only use for a short time until cause of delirium is identified and treated, then discontinue.

No → **See change in intake of food or fluids**

No → **Change in intake of food or fluids?**
(Possible indicators of malnutrition or dehydration)

Yes → **Poor food intake?**

Yes → Check diet preferences, observe ability of patient to feed himself—may need finger foods. Determine if there are dental or oral problems causing inability to chew (tooth decay, poorly fitting dentures, lost dentures). Observe dining setting—too distracting? If so, move to quiet area.

No → **Poor fluid intake?**

Yes → Ensure fluids are available and easy to reach. Ensure fluids are recognizable in transparent containers. Offer small amounts of fluids frequently. Check patient preferences. Check for sore throat. Get medical consult.

No → **Possible pain?**

No → **See possible pain**

Yes → Do body audit to identify possible cause; look for bruising, tight clothing, too many layers, wearing someone else's clothes that don't fit, rumpled sheets causing skin breakdown.

No → **Possible infection?**

Yes → Check vital signs; listen to lungs; review recent lab results; blood sugar.

No → Seek help in finding the cause of delirium.

Figure 2-3 Suggested approach to evaluating cause of delirium.

- Usually occurs early in the course of dementia
- Somatic complaints "My back hurts! I need the doctor!"
- Sleep disturbance (early morning awakening and pacing)
- Appetite disturbance, refusal or decline in eating or drinking)
- Anhedonia, lack of pleasure from usual activities
- Apathy, refusal to get out of bed or get dressed
- Tearfulness

Care of Patients with Depression

DOs	DON'Ts
• Recognize that a change has occurred.	• Think the depression is a result of living in a nursing home and fail to treat the patient.
• Obtain an evaluation by a psychologist/psychiatrist for diagnosis.	• Ignore the changes you see.
• Be supportive! "I am sorry you are feeling low but I'll help you."	• Tell the patient to "get it together!"
• Keep patient active, washed, groomed, and out of bed.	• Allow the patient to stay in bed all day.
• Make sure patients eat even if you have to provide encouragement during meals.	• Allow the patient to refuse food, fluids, and medications.
• Make sure patients get adequate fluids; identify favorites and offer them.	
• Educate the patient's family and other caregivers that this is not just "giving up" but another treatable condition.	

> ### Box 2-4 **Depression Reminders**
>
> - Depression is common and patients suffer because of it.
> - Depression is treatable.
> - Antidepressants take time to work.
> - Patient may need psychiatric admission.
> - Electroconvulsive treatment (ECT) is fast and works.

HALLUCINATIONS

Hallucinations Defined

Hallucinations are a sensory perception without a stimulus. The most common hallucinations seen in dementia patients are visual and auditory.

- Visual hallucinations: Seeing things, animals, persons who are not there
- Auditory hallucinations: Hearing sounds, voices that are not present

More rare types of hallucinations include:

- Olfactory hallucinations: Odd smells
- Gustatory hallucinations: Unusual tastes
- Tactile hallucinations: Feeling things, often things crawling on the skin

  Hallucinations must be distinguished from illusions, which are also common.

Key Observations Indicating Hallucinations

Visual. Patient looks at an area and moves away or seems afraid when nothing is there. Patient points at an empty area of a room and may say "Don't you see it?"

Box 2-5 Hallucinations Versus Illusions

Hallucinations are sensory experiences without a stimulus. Illusions are misperceptions of something that is there, such as thinking people on the television are in the room. In that case, turn off the TV!

When a patient experiences an illusion, something in the environment is upsetting. Try to find and eliminate the aspect of the environment that upsets the patient:

- Reduce clutter

- Eliminate shadows

- Eliminate glare on windows

- Close the blinds

- Remove mirrors

Auditory. Patient looks to side and has conversation when no one is present

Olfactory. Patient complains "I smell a dead animal in here!"

Gustatory. Patient spits out food, complains that something is wrong in his or her mouth, or that the food is spoiled or rotten

Care of Patients with Hallucinations

DOs	DON'Ts
• Directly ask the patient "Do you see someone or something that is upsetting you?"	• Argue with the patient, such as saying, "There is nothing there! Just calm down!"

- Distract the patient and move him or her to another room or go for a walk.
- Reassure the patient by saying you don't see anything, but you are sorry he or she is upset. Offer to help.
- If patient is suffering or the hallucinations prevent you from providing adequate care, tell the charge nurse or doctor. Hallucinations are common in delirium and must be treated. Medications must be reviewed as they are a common cause of hallucinations.
- Treat with antipsychotic medications, if necessary.

- Attempt to reason with the patient.
- Ignore this symptom; hallucinations must be reported and evaluated.
- Force a patient into a situation he or she perceives as frightening.
- Tell the patient he or she is imagining things.

Box 2-6 What to Say to Patients with Hallucinations

The primary response to patients who hallucinate should be one of concern for their safety and comfort. Example: A female patient with dementia won't go into the shower room. You take her in and ask "What is upsetting you?" She says "I won't take my clothes off in front of all those men!" (There is no one else present.) Although the patient is hallucinating, respond to her perceived discomfort. Say, "Let's leave and come back later, don't worry, I'll make sure you are safe." Switch gears and wash the patient at the sink in her room or attempt the shower later.

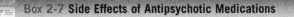

Box 2-7 **Side Effects of Antipsychotic Medications**

Antipsychotic medications can have serious side effects:

- Orthostatic hypotension (sudden drop in blood pressure when standing)

- Stiffness

- Shuffling gait

- Masked facies

- Drowsiness

- Delirium

- Dizziness

Patients on these medications must be carefully monitored and side effects reported promptly!

DELUSIONS

Delusions Defined

Delusions consist of fixed false beliefs. Most common are suspicious ideas to which the patient tirelessly clings.

Key Observations Indicating Delusions

Patients with delusions will typically make comments based on false beliefs, such as:

- "You stole my sweater!"
- "I have to go home now to feed my children!"
- "I have been abandoned."

- "My husband is unfaithful."
- "I am being held prisoner. Call the police!"

Care of Patients with Delusions

DOs	DON'Ts
• Support the patient and provide comfort.	• Argue or attempt to reason with patients.
• Attempt to distract the patient with walking, food, music, conversation about something else.	• Tell patients they have "crazy ideas."
• Document when and where it happens, to identify patterns and triggers.	• Talk about patients in their presence, as your comments may be misinterpreted.
• Say, "I will help you find your sweater," even though this belief is a delusion.	• Make a joke of patient comments.
• Say, "Let's make a snack for your children." (Telling lies can reduce suffering!)	• Whisper around patients.
• If the patient is at risk because of a false belief, such as someone who tries to break a glass window to get away, get help to keep the person safe.	• Laugh at them.
• Report to charge nurse or doctor for evaluation and diagnosis.	
• If antipsychotic medications are prescribed, monitor side effects carefully.	

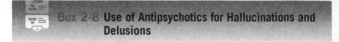

Box 2-8 Use of Antipsychotics for Hallucinations and Delusions

• Avoid prn or as needed dosing.

• Avoid changing type of medication frequently, as side effects from one will not clear rapidly and will accumulate.

• Avoid restraints; they make patients worse.

• Have family members stay with the patient or hire a sitter to stay.

Box 2-9 How to Respond to Patients with Delusions

Enter the patient's world and respond from a perspective that will diffuse the tension and anxiety caused by the delusion. For example, the patient with dementia won't sit to eat because she is looking for her parents who are deceased.

Good response: I'll watch for them while you get started eating. Don't worry, I am sure they are fine and may visit tomorrow.

Poor response: Your parents aren't coming. They would have to be 120 years old. You know they are dead. Stop being uncooperative!

MANIA

Mania Defined

Mania is rare in persons with dementia, but when present it causes significant care challenges. Manic patients are at risk of harm from others if they get physically close, speak to, or touch other people.

Common features of mania:

• State of increased mood or euphoria

• Less need for sleep and food

• Overactivity, talking too much too quickly

- Increased sense of self-importance: "I am the King"
- Irritability
- Hypersexuality, inappropriately touching others, staff or peers
- Getting too close to others, invading their personal space

Care of Manic Patients

DOs	DON'Ts
• Keep the patient safe.	• Laugh at the patient.
• Ensure the patient gets rest.	• Allow the patient to walk for long periods.
• Provide finger foods if patient won't sit down to eat.	• Allow the patient to refuse food or drink.
• Give the patient space and monitor him or her.	• Allow the patient to refuse medications. (If so, be creative and go back again.)
• If antipsychotics or mood stabilizers are given, carefully monitor for side effects.	

APATHY

Apathy Defined

- Lack of initiative and motivation in things the patient previously enjoyed
- Described as "bumps on a log"
- Example: When a patient refuses to participate in the day program

Care of Apathetic Patients

DOs	DON'Ts
• Get patients going with energy and positive statements.	• Allow patients to lie in bed all day.
	• Ignore the apathy.

- Rather than asking "Do you want to go to activities?" just take the patient to activities, saying "Let's have fun."
- Evaluate for depression.
- Evaluate for delirium.
- Evaluate hearing and vision.
- Prevent deconditioning

- Tell patients it is their choice to do nothing.
- Let patients "fall through the cracks" because they are quiet.
- Let patients stay immobile.

REFERENCES

1. Frick DM, Agostini JV, Inouye SK. Delirium superimposed on dementia: a systematic review. *J Am Geriatr Soc* 2002;50: 1723-1732.
2. Lyketsos CG, Steele C, Baker L, et al. Major and minor depression in Alzheimer disease: prevalence and impact. *J Neuropsychiatry Clin Neurosci* 1997;9:556-561.
3. Paulsen JS, Salmon DP, Thal LJ, Romero R. Incidence of and risk factors for hallucinations and delusions in patients with probable AD. *Neurology* 2000;54:1965-1971.
4. Lyketsos CG, Corazzini K, Steele C. Mania in Alzheimer disease. *J Neuropsychiatry Clin Neurosci* 1995;7;350-352.
5. Lyketsos CG, Lopez O, Jones B. Fitzpatrick A, Breitner J, Dekosky S. Prevalence of neuropsychiatric symptoms in dementia and mild cognitive impairment. *JAMA* 2002;288:1475-1483.
6. Inouye SK. Delirium in hospitalized elderly patients: recognition, evaluation and management. *Conn Med* 1993;57:309-315.

Chapter 3

ASSESSMENT— THE VITAL SIGNS of DEMENTIA

Cynthia D. Steele

🔑 Key Points

- Special issues in assessing persons with dementia
- Domains of assessment
- Conducting the Mental Status Examination
- Other assessment tools

IMPORTANCE OF ASSESSMENT

Assessing the patient with dementia is an essential part of appropriate care planning. The effective nurse must know each patient's impairments in thinking and functioning and the severity of each deficit. There are no generic dementia patients, so an accurate assessment allows the nurse to plan specifically for each individual. In addition, assessment data is closely related to the determination of the level of care a patient may receive in terms of reimbursement eligibility.

The nurse will find that changes in both physical and mental functioning are perceptible. Due to the fragile relationship between physical and mental health, the first sign of an emerging medical illness is often a change in mental status. Such is the case with a person suffering a severe depression who is refusing to eat or drink.

Most patients will experience complications of dementia, which result in a change of function, as seen in Figure 3-1. Such changes alert the nurse to conduct a reassessment of the patient to determine the cause and possible treatments.

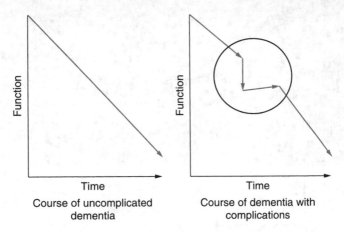

Figure 3-1   Course of uncomplicated and complicated dementia.

SPECIAL ISSUES

Be aware of the special issues in assessing persons with dementia.

- Most patients lack insight into their impairments and will deny anything is wrong. Informants, such as family members or a close friend, must supply critical information.
- Direct testing of cognition is necessary, though many patients consider an assessment of mental abilities as intrusive and embarrassing.
- Because patients cannot describe how they feel, observation and direct questioning are essential.

DOMAINS OF ASSESSMENT

In order to make the assessment comprehensive, the dementia patient must be evaluated from several domains (see Figure 3-2). These domains include:

- Mental status
- Cognition

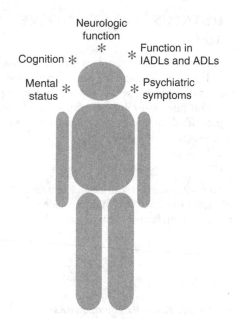

Figure 3-2   Domains of assessment.

- Neurologic function
- Function in Instrumental Activities of Daily Living (IADLs) and Activities of Daily Living (ADLs)
- Psychiatric symptoms

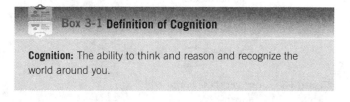

Box 3-1 Definition of Cognition

Cognition: The ability to think and reason and recognize the world around you.

MENTAL STATUS AND COGNITIVE ASSESSMENT

Cognitive impairment or impairment in memory and other functions, such as using language and reasoning, is the hallmark of dementia. As each patient will have his or her own profile of impairments and rate of decline, the nurse should assess and measure a patient's decline *over time* to provide the best possible care at all stages.

Standardized Assessments

There are many standardized scales for assessment of cognition. The Mental Status Examination (MSE) provides a *comprehensive* assessment of mental facility. This is crucial in dementia, as

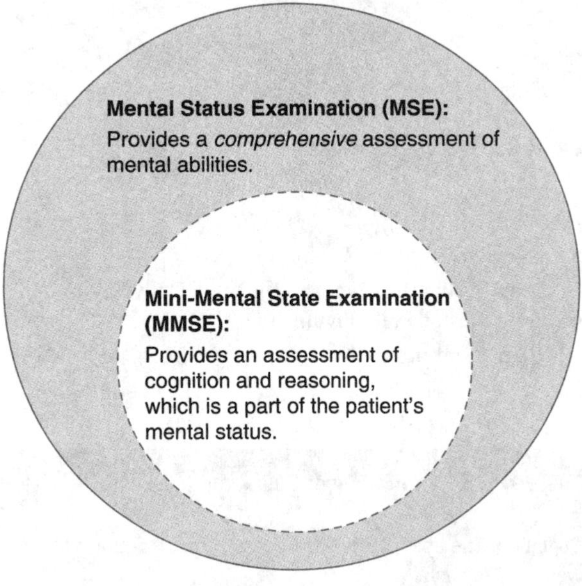

Mental Status Examination (MSE):
Provides a *comprehensive* assessment of mental abilities.

Mini-Mental State Examination (MMSE):
Provides an assessment of cognition and reasoning, which is a part of the patient's mental status.

Figure 3-3   Don't get these confused!

there can be a decline in multiple mental abilities. As part of the overall comprehensive assessment, the Mini-Mental State Examination (MMSE)[1] is often used to assess cognitive ability. Please note that the Mini-Mental State Examination is an assessment of cognition and reasoning, but is not a comprehensive measure of mental status (see Figure 3-3).

Mental Status Examination

The Mental Status Examination (MSE) assesses the patient in six areas listed here.

1. Level of consciousness
2. Appearance and behavior
3. Mood
4. Speech and language
5. Perceptions and beliefs
6. Cognition

Conducting the Mental Status Examination

As the Mental Status Examination will be unfamiliar and in many cases deemed intrusive and embarrassing, special approaches are required to successfully obtain data. Follow these guidelines:

• The examination must be done in private where no one else can hear. Do not conduct the assessment in common areas such as hallways in a nursing facility or hospital.

• To request permission to conduct the MSE, the interviewer should ask directly, "May I speak with you?" and ask, "How are you are feeling?"

• Ensure that the environment is comfortable, quiet, and private.

• Have tissues available and see that the patient has been toileted.

• Use a script and fill in the blank form so nothing is overlooked. See the Appendix for a Mental Status Examination script.

Table 3-1   Normal and Abnormal Levels of Consciousness

Normal Level	Abnormal Level
Awake and alert	Drowsy
Ability to sustain attention	Difficult to sustain attention
Stable consciousness	Fluctuating consciousness—awake and alert one minute and drowsy or asleep the next

To conduct a full Mental Status Examination, evaluate the following areas described here.

Level of consciousness

This is the awareness a person has of his or her environment. Persons with dementia are normally awake and alert during the day and asleep at night. Level of consciousness, as described in Table 3-1, should not fluctuate.

Appearance and behavior

Note the general appearance of the patient, including grooming and dress. These should be appropriate to the age, weather, culture, and ethnic background. Of note: persons with dementia may layer clothes, wear insufficient clothing in the winter, and look unshaven and unkempt. The nurse should observe and record the following:

- Whether or not the patient makes eye contact
- Excess of movement—manifested by those who cannot sit still or continually try to get up and leave an area
- Abnormal tics (repetitive involuntary movements), such as jerking or grunting
- Psychomotor retardation—sitting motionlessly, lacking the normal gestures of communication, often seen in patients who are depressed, or in some cases overmedicated
- Facial expression—pay attention to features such as furrowing the brow
- Body posture and position in regard to the nurse

Box 3-2 Example of Behavior Observations

A manic patient will often sit too close to the nurse and invade his or her personal space. Suspicious patients will often try to avoid sitting close to the interviewer, and may avoid looking directly at the interviewer when answering questions.

Mood

Mood is the third area to be assessed. Mood is a sustained emotional state. Examples of mood states include depression, elation, and anger. Mood should be consistent with the topic of conversation. An example of an inconsistent mood would be observed when a patient laughs at sad topics and cries at pleasant ones. The nurse must ask directly about mood state.

Box 3-3 Important Terms

Depression: A low mood.

Delusion: A fixed, false belief.

Hallucination: A sensory perception in the absence of a stimulus. Examples include hearing voices and seeing things that are not present. Can occur in any of the five senses, but visual hallucinations are most common in persons with dementia.

Illusion: A misperception of things in the patient's environment. An example would be if a patient sees a blanket draped over a chair in a dimly lit room and perceives this as a person looking at the patient.

Speech and language
Speech and language are observed next. Note the patient's rate and rhythm of speech. It is important to observe whether the patient offers spontaneous speech or only answers direct questions. Patients with Alzheimer disease will produce vague and "empty" speech, often lacking nouns. Write down an example of the patient's speech.

Perceptions and beliefs
Perceptions and beliefs are assessed to identify any that are abnormal, which may indicate hallucinations or delusions. Delusions are fixed, false beliefs. In dementia, paranoid or suspicious delusions are most common. An example would be a patient who is convinced that his or her spouse is having an affair or that the food is poisoned. Such patients will often have angry arguments with their spouse and may refuse to eat food.

Cognition
Cognition is broadly defined as the ability to think and reason. Alzheimer disease patients will have global cognitive impairments, including impairments in memory, reasoning, and understanding language. Patients with dementia will make poor decisions and may be disoriented to person, place, and time.

While many cognition assessments are available, the most widely used is the Mini-Mental State Examination (MMSE). This short scale is a screen for cognitive impairment, but not a diagnostic tool. It can be obtained with guidelines for scoring from Psychological Assessment Resources, Inc. The MMSE assesses:

• Orientation to place and time
• Ability to register items in memory
• Concentration
• Comprehension of language
• Recall
• Praxis (ability to execute coordinated movement)
• Ability to follow a multistage command

This assessment is useful for planning care. Also included is the Severe Impairment Rating Scale (SIRS), which assesses more basic functioning. The SIRS is recommended for patients who are too impaired for the Mini-Mental State Examination—those whose score is 5 or less.

Conducting the Mini-Mental State Examination

During the MMSE assessment, ask as few extraneous questions as possible. Rather, ask direct questions, avoiding those that elicit a "yes" or "no" response. Direct questioning will more accurately test a patient's memory.

Do Ask	Don't Ask
What day is it today?	Do you know what day it is?
Where are we now?	Do you know where we are?
What year is it now?	Do you know what year it is?

Box 3-4 Responding during the MMSE

When conducting an MMSE, you will ask the patient a series of questions. Regardless of the patient's response, give positive praise or comments. If an answer is incorrect, do not correct the patient. This will only add to the patient's confusion.

NEUROLOGIC ASSESSMENT

The neurologic examination of the person with dementia is essential, as dementia is a neurologic disease. One must note the neurologic condition of the patient at baseline, as many brain diseases, such as Parkinson disease, have obvious neurologic abnormalities. In addition, many of the medications used in managing behavioral and psychiatric symptoms of dementia result in neurologic impairment.

Box 3-5 Neurologic Terms

Tremor: A repetitive movement of a muscle group that can occur during rest—resting tremor—or while doing something—intention tremor.

Gait: Manner of walking.

Tone: Resting tension in a relaxed muscle.

Akasthisia: The urge to move about; inability to sit still.

Dystonia: Contraction of a muscle that results in an abnormal posture.

- **Observations at rest.** The assessment begins by simply observing the patient at rest, sitting in a chair. Does the patient sit in a normal posture? Are the patient's gestures normal or does he or she sit motionless?
- **Tremors.** Observe *resting tremors*, watching the hands in the lap of the patient. An *intention tremor* can be elicited by asking the patient to reach out the hands as if to stop traffic. Tremors are described as coarse or fine.
- **Gait.** Gait is assessed by asking the patient to walk approximately 3 meters, then to stop, turn around, and walk back. The patient with normal gait stands upright with shoulders over the feet. The patient's steps should not overlap during walking, but rather one foot should precede the other. The individual should pivot as he or she turns.

  In patients with abnormal findings, one will observe that the patient turns "on block," as if made of a block of wood. The patient should not sway during a turn.

  The "get up and go" test is widely used to assess gait. The more abnormal the gait, the higher the risk of a fall. In a normal walk, the arms swing to promote balance. A patient whose arms remain unmoved at his or her side during walking is at high risk for falling.

- **Tone.** Tone is assessed by asking the sitting patient to relax, supporting his or her elbow with your hand and moving the patient's arm through a range of motion. No resistance should be felt.

- **Akasthisia.** Akasthisia is readily observed by watching the patient sitting in a chair. If akasthisia is present, the person will shift about restlessly, unable to sit still. Many patients will express that this urge to move feels uncomfortable. This symptom is also a common side effect of psychotropic medications and an indication that the dose or type of medication should be re-evaluated.

- **Dystonia.** Dystonic postures are extreme and can be a result of high sensitivity to neuroleptic medications. As such, these postures are indicative of an urgent issue that should be dealt with immediately. A call to the attending physician must be made as soon as possible. Dystonic postures, such as when the fingers of the hand are bent backward with the wrist flexed, can be indicative of neuroleptic malignant syndrome, which can be life-threatening.

Box 3-6 Medical Alert: Seriousness of Dystonic Postures

Dystonic postures, sustained muscle contractions that can result in abnormal postures, may be indicative of neuroleptic malignant syndrome, which can be life-threatening.

FUNCTIONAL ASSESSMENT

The ability of the patient to perform both Instrumental Activities of Daily Living (IADLs) and Activities of Daily Living (ADLs) must be assessed, as these abilities will change over time. Gaps in function in these areas must be filled by family or other caregivers.

> **Box 3-7 IADLs and ADLs**
>
> **Instrumental Activities of Daily Living (IADLs)** include the ability to handle money, cook, use transportation, do laundry, manage medications, and use a telephone.
>
> **Activities of Daily Living (ADLs)** include basic tasks such as dressing, feeding, toileting, walking, and bathing.

Instrumental Activities of Daily Living include the ability to handle money, cook, use transportation, do laundry, manage medications, and use a telephone. Such higher-order abilities erode first, and these impairments are often noticed by family when errors such as forgetting to pay a bill or getting lost are made.

In contrast, activities of daily living include more basic tasks such as dressing, feeding, toileting, walking, and bathing. These skills erode next, and often—as in a person with Alzheimer disease—in a slow and gradual fashion. Often parts of a task are recalled but the order in which they must be completed is forgotten. This is the case when a person puts underwear on over clothing. See Figure 3-4 for a typical progression

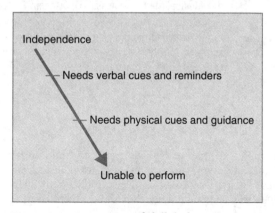

Figure 3-4   Progression of skill decline.

of skill loss. This is the model used in the Psychogeriatric Dependency Rating Scale (PGDRS)[2] and is very useful in constructing detailed care plans.

Please note the review of abilities in IADLs and ADLs must be conducted with someone who knows the patient well. Follow-up phone calls to the informant may be necessary to complete this part of the assessment. Functional assessment is crucial for making decisions about what level of care the patient will require.

PSYCHIATRIC ASSESSMENT

Approximately half of those with dementia will also suffer from an additional psychiatric condition. These include:

- Delirium
- Depression
- Hallucinations
- Delusions
- Mania
- Apathy

Most of these conditions will be identified during the Mental Status Examination described earlier. When psychiatric conditions are identified, the attending physician must be notified in order to assess the need for treatment, such as psychiatric medications and appropriate supportive care.

There are many standardized tests that can be administered both to identify psychiatric conditions and to monitor the condition's response to treatment. Assessments that measure various types of conditions are listed in Table 3-2.

OVERALL ASSESSMENT PLAN

Your clinical team should make an informed decision as to which scales they will use, obtain training to achieve good interrater reliability, and use the same scales over time. For example, we suggest completing the Mini-Mental State Examination

Table 3-2   Summary of Psychiatric Assessments

Assessment Domain	Early to Mid-Stage Illness	Late Stage
Cognition	Mini-Mental Scale	SIRS
Depression	Cornell Scale for Depression in Dementia[3]	
Function IADL	KATZ IADL scale	
Function ADL	PGDRS	

on admission and every 6 months after that, or more frequently if sudden changes occur. A care plan based on clear data obtained in an orderly way will provide a sound foundation for future planning. Because most dementing illnesses are progressive, it is essential to repeat assessments at regular intervals.

Frequency of Assessments

- **On Admission:** Conduct a comprehensive assessment on admission to your care. This will provide the baseline for care planning.
- **Sudden Changes:** When sudden changes in functioning, cognition or behavior occur, repeat the assessments. This data will inform you of how much decline has occurred and allow you to monitor the selected treatment.
- **6-Month Intervals:** Barring sudden changes, conduct assessments every 6 months, including the Mini-Mental State Examination.
- **Red Flags:** Expect a steady decline in cognition and function over time. Note that sudden severe declines are red flags that an additional condition, such as an infection, may be present. In these cases, a thorough investigation is needed.

The availability of assessment data greatly assists the nurse when an attending physician or consultant must be called to help. In addition to the assessments discussed in this chapter, bowel, bladder, and medication records are also a necessity.

REFERENCES

1. Folstein MF, Folstein SE, McHugh PR. Mini-mental state. A practical method for grading the cognitive state of patients for the clinician. *J Psychiatric Res* 1975;12:189-198.
2. Wilkinson IM, Graham-White J. Psychogeriatric dependency rating scales: a method of assessment for use by nurses *Br J Psychiatry* 1980;137:558-565.
3. Alexopoulos GS, Abrams RC, Young RC, Shamolan CA. Cornell scale for depression in dementia, *Biological Psychiatry* 1988; 23:271-85.

Chapter 4

CAREGIVING BASICS

Cynthia D. Steele

🔑 Key Points

- Four-Part Treatment Model as a framework for care
- Essential principles of caregiving
- Adapting the environment for each patient
- Responding to the effects of amnesia, aphasia, apraxia, and agnosia

Patients with dementia require individualized care. The effort spent in getting to know and understand each patient is rewarded in the ability to provide successful care. Individualizing care for each patient can be accomplished by following the Four-Part Treatment Model described here and by applying the essential principles of caregiving discussed later in this chapter.

THE FOUR-PART TREATMENT MODEL

The Four-Part Treatment Model is an organizing principle for providing optimum care to patients. This model facilitates a patient-centered approach to caregiving by viewing the whole patient from a variety of perspectives.

Part I: Treat the Disease (Purview of the Physician)

Conduct a diagnostic evaluation and offer dementia medications if appropriate. This is the job of the physician.

Part II: Treat the Symptoms

In patients with dementia, nurses should focus on all symptoms: cognitive, functional, psychiatric, and behavioral.

- **Cognitive impairments:** Recognize impairments and limitations and support what remains.
- **Functional decline:** Observe what the patient can do and fill the gaps to maximize function.
- **Psychiatric and behavioral problems:** Recognize psychiatric symptoms and disorders and assure appropriate treatment (see Chapter 2).
- Systematically observe and respond to behavioral problems (see Chapter 6).

Part III: Support the Patient

Because of cognitive decline, dementia patients are typically not able to take care of their own safety and physical and mental health. Nurses can support their patients by compensating for this loss in ability.

Assure Safety

- Personal safety: Ensure that the environment is safe (see "Adapting the Environment" later in the chapter).
- Put identification bracelets on the patient before he or she wanders out.
- Establish power of attorney for health care.
- Make sure important possessions are secure so they cannot be lost.
- Do not permit access to food if the patient cannot tell whether the food is spoiled.

Pay Vigilant Attention to Physical Health

- Take inventory of chronic conditions and assure their ongoing treatment.

- Prevent conditions such as flu by assuring that flu shots are administered; keep patients away from ill persons.
- Ensure that a competent individual is administering medications.
- Find all the medications to which the patient has access—have the family look in kitchen drawers, bathrobe pockets, etc.
- Provide proper oral care—have teeth cleaned by a dentist every 3 to 6 months if possible; check to see if dentures fit and examine gums routinely.

Ensure Proper Nutrition

- Provide adequate and appropriate meals in a form that the patient can recognize and eat (see "Eating" in Chapter 5).

Ensure Patients Are Hydrated

- Avoid caffeine.
- Offer fluids every 2 hours. Note that patients often cannot recognize fluids in opaque containers on bedside tables or recognize drinks in the refrigerator.

Provide Engaging Activities

- Provide meaningful and routine activities (see Chapter 7).

Part IV: Support the Caregiver

Caregiver support can be provided through education, guidance, and referrals to community resources.

Provide Education to Families and Patients

- Explain the patient's illness, what dementia means, and how the patient will decline over time.
- Determine what new skills the caregiver must take over from the patient, such as bill paying and cooking.

Provide Guidance in Decision-Making

- Help to determine if the patient should be left alone (a home OT evaluation is very useful).
- Help to determine if the patient should still drive (formal driving evaluations are useful).
- Help to determine if power of attorney should be in effect by assessing if the patient can no longer make sound decisions about money, property, and health care.
- Help to determine when the patient's illness requires care outside the home (see Chapter 10).

Provide Referrals to Community Resources

- Assist each family in identifying appropriate and affordable resources such as adult day care, home care, assisted living, support groups, and nursing homes.

PRINCIPLES OF CAREGIVING

There are essential principles that nurses can apply within the Four-Part Treatment Model to provide patient-centered care.

Box 4-1 Caregiving Basics

- Know the person for whom you are caring.
- Empathize with the patient.
- Be where the patient is.
- Be flexible.
- Focus on the patient first, the task second.
- Recognize impairments and support strengths.
- Communicate effectively.
- Break down tasks.

The underlying concept of all the principles is to understand the person who lives behind the screen of dementia. Nurses must take into account the life story and the needs and feelings of each dementia patient to create an individualized care environment. The basic principles of caregiving for dementia patients are described here.

Know the Patient

There are no generic dementia patients. Understanding key information about each individual allows the nurse to tailor care to the patient's specific needs and wants. For example, some patients enjoy being in groups and others prefer to be alone. Attempting to force all persons into a large group activity will work for some and not for others.

Box 4-2 What to Find Out about Each Person

- How old is the patient?
- Where was the patient born and raised?
- Is the patient single or married? Does he or she have children or grandchildren?
- What was the patient's occupation (include being a mother or homemaker)?
- What did the patient enjoy doing? Painting? Fixing cars?
- What are the patient's usual routines? Is he or she an early riser or a night owl?

Many dementia patients recall their past and are unable to understand or remember the present. Nurses should inquire about each patient's history and current status. Important information about each individual's past will provide bridges for the future. For example, distracting a patient by talking about his or her past can make unpleasant tasks more palatable for the individual.

Box 4-3 **Advantages of Knowing Your Patients**

If you know that a patient spent his or her life farming, you can talk about animals, crops, or other aspects of farm life while you are giving the patient a bath. This not only distracts the patient who may not like to bathe, but provides dignity and respect for who the person was before becoming demented.

Empathy

Empathy is the ability to appreciate what the patient is experiencing—the ability to walk in the patient's shoes. Try to imagine what life would be like if nothing in your environment or experience seemed familiar. Dementia patients usually do not know where they are, they do not know the people around them, and they do they know what to expect. Most important, most dementia patients do not realize there is anything wrong with them or that they need any kind of help. This is not denial but an inability to appreciate their current state as a result of the brain damage of dementia. Thus, persons with dementia may not thank caregivers for their help.

Empathy includes being sensitive to the feelings of the patient. Statements such as "I would be upset too" validate the reality of what the patient is experiencing. Nurses can form a relationship with a dementia patient even if the patient has no ability to remember.

Be Where the Patient Is

It is important to understand that many patients are "living in the past." A common example is an elderly woman who believes she is a young mother and must go to meet the school bus. Some caregivers worry that accepting that fact is "buying into" a false idea. A better approach would be to accept the patient's reality.

In this case, try to encourage the patient to make a snack for the children or inquire how many children the patient has. Remember that the feelings each patient is experiencing are real. Accepting these feelings is essential, whether or not they make sense. Many disputes can be avoided if a nurse recognizes that he or she cannot force the patient into the present.

Be Flexible

Flexibility is one of the most important approaches to dementia care. Many caregivers feel pressured to get things done according to their own schedule. This is especially common in nursing homes and hospitals where the nurse is scheduled to care for several patients. If the patient resists your efforts to get something done, such as being shaved, it is often better to stop and try later. For example, some patients refuse to get dressed before going into the dining room to eat breakfast. Allowing these patients to eat in their pajamas will not hurt them and avoids an unnecessary struggle. Flexibility does not mean the nurse is lazy; rather it means the nurse wisely understands that further attempts to force the patient would be upsetting.

When a patient is resistant, another flexible approach is allowing a different caregiver to attempt the task. Sometimes the distraction of a new face will stop the patient's resistance and allow the task to be completed. This does not mean the first nurse has failed, but rather the nurse found a flexible and better way to accomplish a task.

Communicate Effectively

Communication Impairments

Communication is a two-way street. A message has to be given by one person and understood by another. Most, if not all, dementia patients will have communication impairments. They will have difficulty producing meaningful language and also understanding what is said. The speech of dementia patients may seem "empty" or lacking direction. At the same time, the speech of dementia patients can retain the rhythm and gestures of normal speech even if the words make little sense. Early on, dementia patients lose the ability to remember the names of objects but may be able to describe their function. A common example would be a thirsty patient who has a cup in front of him and says, "I need the thing for drinking."

Body Language and Key Words

Watching body language is a key aspect of effective communication. Patients may be able to point to what they want or push a caregiver away when touching a part of their body causes pain. Remember that behavior is communication. Listening carefully for key words in the middle of seemingly rambling sentences can enable the nurse to know what a patient wants or needs. Some patients are embarrassed by their language difficulties and can become withdrawn as a result. Careful observation of the patient's body language and listening for key words can restore confidence to patients and help them to be more social and functional.

Enhancing Communication

There are many ways that nurses can enhance their end of the communication:

- Make certain the patient knows you are there and can hear you.
- Ensure that hearing aids are in place and functional.
- Assure eyeglasses and clean and in place on the patient.
- Make eye contact with the patient.
- Speak slowly, using simple words.
- Use a low tone of voice.
- Raising your voice when the patient does not understand the words will make matters worse.
- When words fail, use gestures such as gentle physical guidance.
- Mirror behaviors that you want to encourage.

  Show them what you want them to do by doing it yourself in front of them.

Box 4-4 **Mirroring**

The "mirroring" technique can enhance a nurse's ability to communicate with patients who have communication impairments. The technique involves demonstrating the behavior you would like the patient to perform. For example, instead of taking a resistant patient to the dining room and saying "Go sit in your seat," you could mirror sitting. Simply pull out a chair next to where the patient should sit, sit down, and say "Join me."

Clearly there are times when words only upset a patient who cannot understand. In this situation, just moving through a task, such as dressing silently and slowly, is the best option. It is essential that only one person speaks to the patient at a time. If a task such as dressing or bathing takes two caregivers, they must decide before approaching the patient who will speak to the patient and who will do the care. Who will be the "doer" and who will be the "talker."

Is There a Place for Lying?

The issue of lying to a dementia patient causes a struggle for most nurses. Lying to an adult may feel uncomfortable or wrong. An impact of the memory loss as a result of dementia results in patients repeating the same questions and insisting that false things are true. The brain disease causing dementia prevents patients from appreciating and accepting the truth. Insisting that they do often leads to increased distress in both the patient and caregiver. Try to distract the patient or focus on his or her feelings—this allows the patient to know that he or she is heard, and enhances the relationship between caregiver and patient. When distraction or acknowledging the patient's feelings does not calm the individual, lying seems justifiable. The goal of lying is to relieve distress.

Box 4-5 Communication Tips

Understanding the Patient

- Listen for key words.
- Observe body language and try to understand it.

Communicating to the Patient

- Assure that the patient can see and hear you.
- Be at eye level with the patient; kneel down if necessary.
- Eliminate other distractions such as TV and radio—close the door of the room.
- Do not talk from behind or beside the patient.
- Use simple language.
- Allow the patient time to respond; be patient.
- Use a low tone of voice; don't yell.
- Have only one person talking at a time to the patient.
- Use gestures and actions that the patient can "mirror."
- If words confuse and upset the patient, don't use them.

Box 4-6 Addressing the Patient

An issue of concern for many nurses is how to address the patient. In normal circumstances, one would be formal and call a patient Mr. ___ or Mrs. ___. But many patients have forgotten their formal names and do not respond to them. Also, many married women remember only their maiden names or just their first names. Families can tell you what name the patient responds to and give you permission to use it.

Be cautious about using terms of endearment such as "Honey" or "Sweetheart." Such terms can be misinterpreted by patients and in some cases provoke behavior in kind (e.g., the case of an elderly man who is called "sweetheart" and responds by reaching for the breasts of the caregiver).

Box 4-7 Responding to a Patient's False Beliefs

When an 85-year-old dementia patient insists that her mother and father are alive, the proper first responses include distraction, such as "Let's go get the dining room ready," and acknowledging the patient's feelings: "It seems you miss your parents." Unfortunately, such tactics don't always calm the patient. When these approaches do not relieve the patient's distress, try to accommodate the patient's reality by saying something like, "Let's get dressed in case they come to visit you" or "Yes, your parents love you very much." Attempting to make the patient face the blunt truth, "Your parents are dead," is not only useless but escalates the patient's discomfort.

In addition, lying to a patient can be very useful in accomplishing tasks that upset the patient, such as bathing or showering. When distraction and validation of feelings fail, a supportive statement, such as "Let's get ready for a visit from family," will often facilitate getting through the task. By the time the task is over, many dementia patients will have forgotten they were told their family was visiting.

Focus on the Patient First, the Task Second

Approaching the patient with a smile and social greeting before attempting care can enhance cooperation. Walking into a room and saying "Good morning, we're going to have a good day today" instead of saying "Time to get up and dressed now" will be more successful. It is prudent to always let the patient know who you are, as dementia patients forget even if you care for them every day. Saying "I am Susan, your helper today" also sets up proper boundaries. Pausing after a social greeting allows the patient to get used to your presence before you attempt to touch him of her. Speaking first and touching second is always better.

Recognize Impairments and Support Strengths

Gradual Loss of Ability

Dementia patients gradually lose the ability to perform daily tasks. They can often complete part of a task but need help at certain steps (e.g., a patient who can brush his or her teeth if you put toothpaste on the brush and hand it to the patient). It is the nurse's responsibility to fill the gaps and allow the person to do as much as possible. Remember that abilities will decline over time, and it will be necessary to give more help as the disease progresses. If it seems the patient is not trying, he or she may have progressed beyond the ability to perform the task.

Low Periods

It is also true that patients can do more on some days than others and will need additional help during the low periods. This variation in function is often misinterpreted as a lack of cooperation, but is more likely a result of something else such as lack of sleep or sensory overload at the time. It is important to communicate when a patient is having a "low period" or "bad day" so that co-workers do not become frustrated with the patient.

Praise and Encouragement

When going through the steps of an activity such as dressing, it is important to offer praise for what the patient *can* do. For example, if a patient can put his arm in a sleeve, it is good to say, "Good job" and be encouraging.

Task Breakdown

Most of what we do in a normal day involves many steps that seem automatic to us. Getting out of a chair involves moving your body forward over your feet, grabbing the arms of the chair, pushing up, and standing. Although we don't think about these automatic tasks, dementia patients often need guidance and prompting to perform each step. It is important to understand how many steps a patient can perform independently and how many steps need to be prompted.

ADAPTING THE ENVIRONMENT

In support of the Four-Part Treatment Model, the nurse can contribute a great deal by ensuring that the environment is adapted to the patient's individual needs. Most dementia patients move through a variety of environments, beginning at home and eventually moving to long-term care facilities. In the early stages, patients may be home with a caregiver. Often this care is supplemented by adult day care. If the caregiver is absent or no longer able to provide the care, many persons move to assisted living facilities during the middle stages. These facilities range from small homes accommodating 5 or fewer persons to large commercial chains with 15 to 100 or more beds. Nursing homes are often the final environment for patients in late-stage dementia. The basic principles of adaptation of the environment can be applied to any setting and are summarized here:

Key Aspects of the Adapted Environment

The ideal environment for a patient with dementia is simple and uncluttered. The environment should be:

1. Familiar—a bedroom should look like a bedroom, a dining room should look like a dining room, and a bathroom should look familiar as well.
2. Safe—free of obstacles such as low furniture, throw rugs, access to sharp objects, medications, stoves, and unsecured stairways.
3. Quiet—free of overhead paging, constant television, or radio.
4. Enhanced by cues—good visual access to bathrooms for easy identification and free of miscues such as hats and coats, which prompt patients to want to leave.

CAREGIVING AND THE FOUR A'S

The primary symptoms of dementia are the 4 A's:

- Amnesia: Memory impairment
- Aphasia: Communication impairment

- Apraxia: Impairment in performing motor movements
- Agnosia: Impairment in recognition of what is taken in through the senses

Although each symptom causes impairments for the patient, there are effective ways to respond to each symptom.

Amnesia: Impact on the Patient

Patients with amnesia often experience the following impairments:

- Cannot form new memories
- May insist dead relatives are alive
- Will lose their things and accuse others of stealing
- Will stop in the midst of a task, forgetting the steps
- Will not remember how to use the call bell
- Will not remember they cannot get out of bed without assistance
- Will not remember to use assistive devices like walkers or canes
- Repeat questions numerous times

Amnesia: The Response

Suggested responses to patients experiencing amnesia are:

- Do not expect or rely on the patient to remember.
- Do not get irritated when a patient cannot remember.
- If a patient insists dead relatives are alive, just "be with them" and ask about the relatives; try to distract the patient.
- Have empathy; "I'm sorry you can't find your sweater, I'll help you find it."
- Use task breakdown, giving directions one step at a time.
- Check on patients frequently as they won't call for assistance but may attempt to find something or someone familiar by wandering out.
- Remove cues from the environment. If you don't want the patient to get up, do not have a coat and hat visible.

• If a patient repeats questions, acknowledge the patient, but don't say "I just told you." Sometimes not replying is best.

Aphasia: Impact on the Patient

Patients with aphasia often experience the following impairments:

• Will not remember names of things
• Become frustrated when they cannot get you to understand
• Say "yes" when they mean "no"
• Will not understand your directions even though they can hear you
• Become upset with many persons talking simultaneously, and in noisy environments such as dining rooms

Aphasia: The Response

Suggested responses to patients experiencing aphasia are:

• Move the patient to a quiet environment to enhance communication.
• Gain attention of patient before speaking.
• Position your body at eye level with patients.
• Speak slowly and simply.
• Do not raise your voice.
• Use gestures.
• Observe body language of patients to try to understand what they want or need.
• Listen for key words.
• One person should talk at a time.

Apraxia: Impact on the Patient

Patients with apraxia often experience the following impairments:

• Will not be able to do motor tasks such as dressing and using utensils to eat
• May have difficulty in sitting down in a chair, or getting into and out of a bed or car

- May fall
- May not be able to open containers of food on a tray
- May not be able to step into a shower

Apraxia: The Response

Suggested responses to patients experiencing apraxia are:

- Simplify clothing.
- Open containers of food for them.
- Gently guide them to sit safely.
- To get into a chair, back the patient up so the backs of the patient's legs touch the chair, guide your hand down to the patient's arm, and guide the patient down.
- Use task breakdown, assisting where necessary and letting patients do the steps they can (for example, give the patient a washcloth to hold in the shower even though you must wash her).

Agnosia: Impact on the Patient

Patients with agnosia often experience the following impairments:

- Will not recognize the world around them
- Wander around trying to find something familiar
- Rummage in drawers (theirs or others) looking for something that is "lost"
- May not recognize food as edible and may eat anything
- May not recognize their own reflection in a mirror
- May think that persons in pictures or on TV are really there

Agnosia: The Response

Suggested responses to patients experiencing agnosia are:

- Try to make the environment as familiar as possible.
- Eliminate as much clutter as possible.

- If upset by their reflection in the mirror, cover it or take it down.
- If upset by pictures, remove them; turn off the TV and radio.
- Make sure the environment is "dementia safe" (don't put things that patients might eat on medical carts, or counters; secure cleaning carts and supplies).

Chapter 5

COMMON PROBLEMS in DAILY CARE

Cynthia D. Steele

🔑 Key Points

- Planning for daily care activities
- Common difficulties associated with daily care
- Solutions to difficulties with daily care

This chapter will review common challenges in providing daily care to dementia patients. Problems increase from early to middle to late-stage disease. Early in the illness, simply placing objects into view may be all that is needed to prompt a patient to care for himself or herself. As the disease progresses, verbal and physical cues will be needed to initiate the patient to action. During late-stage illness, all daily care may need to be done by the caregiver.

Even though there are distinctions in symptom profiles for different types of dementia, care strategies are basically similar

---

Box 5-1 Tips for Activities of Daily Living

- Keep things simple.
- Always consider what the patient can do and where the gaps need to be filled.
- Be social first and task-centered second.
- Plan a task before beginning it.

across types. Many of the root causes of difficulties in activities of daily living are in the disease impairments themselves. Solutions will be suggested, and as always, they must be tried and modified to suit the individual situation.

GENERAL GUIDELINES

Prior to approaching a patient to accomplish tasks of daily care, make a plan of how you will complete the task. Follow these guidelines to be most effective.

- Gather all supplies you will need before beginning.
- If it will take more than one person to complete the task, decide who will talk to the patient and how others will assist.
- Allow only one person to speak to the patient at a time. More than that may confuse and frighten the patient.
- Be social first and task-centered second. When approaching a patient, smile and greet the patient. Introduce yourself—do not assume the patient can remember who you are.
- Make sure the patient is paying attention to you before you begin. That is, make sure a patient can see you and hear you before touching the patient.
- Speak to the patient at eye level; do not stand above the patient.

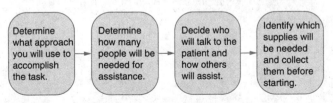

Figure 5-1   Planning an activity of daily living.

> **Box 5-2 Avoiding Conflict**
>
> Remember these types of phrases can help avoid confrontations with patients who are triggered by tasks of daily living.
>
> • If the word "bath" or "shower" upsets the patient, just say, "Let's go get freshened up," or simply "Come along with me."
> • If a protective cloth is required during eating, do not call it a "bib." Tell the patient, "This will keep you warm and dry."
> • Rather than asking a contrary patient who is on a toileting schedule to go to the bathroom, simply hold out your arm and say "Let's go for a walk."

DRESSING

There are many possible causes of difficulties with dressing for the dementia patient.

Possible Causes of Dressing Problems

- Inability to choose from the many options of clothing in the closet
- Inability to remember where things are if they are not in direct view
- Forgetting the proper order for putting on clothes
- Getting easily distracted
- Impairment in fine-motor skills, making fasteners, zippers, and buttons difficult to use
- Embarrassment due to lack of privacy in a facility
- A room that is too cold
- Being rushed by a caregiver
- Inability to select appropriate clothing for the weather or occasion

- Lack of ability to tell soiled clothing from clean clothing
- Wanting to wear the same clothes every day

Solutions to Dressing Problems

General Guidelines

- Limit choices.
- If the patient resides in a group setting, label all clothing.
- It is often helpful to dress the top half of the body first, assisting as needed. Caregiver assistance should start with holding out the item.

Encourage Independence

- Allow patients to do as much as they can by themselves.
- If patients can still dress themselves, put one outfit in view. If they need cueing for the order of dressing, hold out one item at a time, oriented properly to the body.
- At times, getting a patient started—such as putting a hand into a sleeve—will activate the process.
- Provide praise for each step completed.

Insistence on Wearing the Same Clothes

- If patients insist on wearing the same clothing each day, order sets of identical clothing and have only a clean set within reach and view.
- It may be necessary to go into the patient's room when he or she is not present and remove soiled clothing, replacing it with clean clothing.

Patients Who Cannot Dress Themselves

- In some cases it is helpful to wash the patient in bed and begin the dressing task there.
- One approach is to change the underwear and slide on pants or slacks to the knees, put on socks and shoes while the patient is lying down, then sit the patient up to dress the

upper body. Quickly pull up pants/slacks and stand the patient up. This prevents the patient from kicking at you while trying to put on shoes and socks.

Special Situations

* If a patient repeatedly tries to undress in public, assess the patient to see if the clothing no longer fits or is uncomfortable. For these patients, make clothing harder to get off by using a buttoned shirt rather than one that pulls on over the head.
* One-piece jumpsuits are available, as some patients with a need to use the bathroom cannot ask where it is and may attempt to disrobe in public.
* Observing someone routinely fidgeting with their clothing will clue the caregiver to the need to escort the patient to the bathroom and assist in toileting.

Box 5-3 Quick Tips for Dressing

* Limit the clothing choices.
* Encourage patients to remain independent.
* When needed, cue patients by handing them one piece of clothing at a time.
* When needed, initiate dressing by getting the patient started.
* Provide lots of praise.

BATHING

Bathing and showering are some of the most difficult tasks to be accomplished with the dementia patient. It is this task, more than any other, that places the staff at risk for combative behavior by the patient. There are many reasons for struggles in bathing, and creativity is essential.

Possible Causes of Bathing Problems

- It is an intimate task that is embarrassing to the patient.
- Institutional bathrooms do not look familiar to the patient and may be frightening.
- The sound of the water, which many patients cannot see, may be frightening.
- In many situations, the patient must be undressed before bathing, thus making the patient cold.
- If the bathroom is all one color, such as white, the patient may have difficulty seeing the tub and resist stepping in due to a fear of falling. Place a colorful contrasting mat inside the tub.

Possible Solutions to Bathing Difficulties

General Guidelines

- Keep it simple. Become familiar with the patient's usual routine. Bath or shower? Morning or evening? Assure privacy.
- Have clean clothing and all supplies in the bath or shower, but keep clean clothing out of sight as it may cue the patient to dress rather than undress.
- Make sure the room is warmed prior to taking the patient into the bathroom.
- Put a bench and grab bars in the bathing area.
- Put a bath blanket over the patient to respect the person's privacy during undressing.
- Allow the patient to do as much as he or she can. If the patient resists having a caregiver take off his or her clothes, provide something to hold, such as a washcloth or a preferred food, for distraction.

Accommodate Impairments

- If the word "bath" or "shower" upsets the patient, just say "Let's go get freshened up" or simply "Come along with me." Remember, lying or not telling the whole truth can be merciful and greatly assist in getting through difficult tasks.

- If the patient seems frightened to step into a tub with water because he or she cannot see it, use bath foam.
- For the patient who fights going into the shower or tub room, try providing a bed bath. Be sure to keep the patient warm and covered. This can be a pleasant alternative. In a double room, pull the curtain or close the door.
- When bathing a patient who is very aphasic, it may be more effective to just carry out the tasks of daily care than to use a lot of language and directions the patient cannot understand.
- Many new products are available to assist with bathing. One is a bag of wipes that can be placed in a microwave to keep them warm. Some cleansing agents do not require rinsing, thus eliminating an upsetting step. Shower caps with shampoo in them can be placed on the patient's head and gently manipulated to clean hair.
- Although a bath with a frightened patient may take all morning, the primary goal is to get the job done without upsetting the individual.
- If a patient strongly resists or strikes out at you, stop the task and try later. Sometimes having an assistant outside the room, who pretends to come in and save the patient, can sufficiently distract the person so that the bath can be completed.
- Holding a patient down during bathing will only result in further struggle. The more upset the patient gets, the calmer the caregiver should be.

Box 5-4 Quick Tips for Bathing

- Protect the patient's privacy.
- Try to accommodate the patient's previous routine.
- Alleviate the fear of falling by making the area safe.
- Encourage independence.
- Have clean clothes close at hand.

EATING

Mealtime challenges are an especially important issue in nursing facilities where the majority of residents are demented. Those who are demented are at higher risk for dehydration and malnutrition for many reasons.

Possible Causes for Mealtime Challenges

- Patients lose the ability to recognize food as something edible.
- Patients lose the ability to use utensils.
- Patients are frequently distracted by the noise and activity in busy dining rooms.
- Patients may be overwhelmed by busy trays with covers over plates and cups. They don't know how to open unfamiliar containers and recognize that food is within the containers. Such patients may get up and leave the table due to frustration.
- Eventually, patients forget how to chew and swallow.

In Early Stages

- Patients may forget to eat.
- Patients may become distracted and leave the table before finishing.

In Middle Stages

- Patients may lack the stamina to sit long enough to finish a meal.
- Patients may not understand how to eat.
- Patients may require calorie-dense foods due to restlessness and frequent wandering away from the table.

In Late Stages

- Patients may be unable to distinguish between food and other objects.
- Patients may lack the coordination to chew and swallow.

Special Problems in Long-Term Care Settings

- Staff must often feed several residents and are under pressure to finish before the food gets cold. This results in a "task-oriented" rather than "person-oriented" approach.
- Longer time to chew and swallow makes feeding take much longer.
- Poor oral health, dentures that don't fit, and mouth pain may result in food refusal.
- When patients lose weight, they are often offered supplements between meals that will diminish appetite at mealtime.
- Dining areas are often cluttered, noisy, and chaotic.
- Staff member changes often interfere with the individual understanding how a patient eats and what his or her preferences are.

Possible Solutions for Mealtime Challenges

General Guidelines

- Adhere to mealtime routines—have the patient sit at the same chair and provide the same dining staff, when possible.
- Understand former preferences and mealtime rituals (example: some will not eat without a prayer).
- Maximize vision and hearing—put clean glasses and hearing aids on the patient.
- Ensure that staff is aware of choking risks and review emergency procedures with staff.
- Avoid garnishes that are not safe to eat.
- If a patient refuses to believe that he or she does not need to pay, issue meal tickets marked "Paid."

Accommodate Small Appetites

- Offer more frequent small meals for those who fatigue during regular meals.
- Keep healthy snacks visible and available.

- Maximize the amount of food provided at the time the patient is most likely to eat. Some patients eat their largest meal at breakfast.

Create a Pleasant Mealtime Environment

- Assure adequate lighting.
- Minimize noise by turning off television; remind staff to not converse among one another at mealtime.
- During meals, chat with the patients about social themes, their early lives, and what their mother cooked, to keep the process going.
- Smile and make meals a social occasion.

Patients Who Need Assistance

- Cut food into bite-sized pieces before presenting to the patient, to preserve dignity.
- When feeding a patient, sit alongside, rather than standing over, the patient.
- If choking is evident, get a swallowing evaluation from an occupational therapist who may suggest the use of thickeners. Thick liquids are easier to swallow than thin ones.
- When feeding a patient, keep him or her in an upright position with head tilted forward.
- Put one item before the patient at a time on a plate with a contrasting placemat.
- Cue as needed, using simple language such as "chew" and "swallow."
- Offer fluids between bites of food to facilitate swallowing and hydration.
- Use hand-over-hand cueing—that is, put your hand over the patient's hand and bring food to the patient's mouth.
- Put hot cereal or soup in a mug.
- If a protective cloth is required, do not call it a "bib." Say, "This will keep you warm and dry."

- When utensils are no longer recognized, use finger foods—make anything into a sandwich.
- If a patient prefers sweets, use a small spoon and put a sweet substance on the tip of the spoon.

Box 5-5 **Quick Tips for Mealtime**

- Maintain mealtime routines.
- Maintain a pleasant environment in the dining area.
- Minimize noise in the dining area.
- Ensure patients have enough food during the time they are most likely to eat.
- Provide finger foods to patients who need assistance.
- Keep the table setting simple so that patients do not get confused.

AMBULATION

Eventually all dementia patients will be unable to walk. This skill erodes over time. Cognitive impairment alone is a strong risk factor for falls, and patients must be observed vigilantly due to the increased risk of falls.

- Difficulties with walking in dementia patients occur due to apraxia. The brain gradually loses the ability to coordinate walking.

Box 5-6 **Common Gaits in Persons with Dementia**

- Shuffling (feet do not lift far above the floor and the feet overlap)
- Swaying gait (broad-based and unsteady)
- Inability to initiate walking when brought to a standing position

Possible Causes of Ambulation Difficulties

- In early stages, walkers and canes can be helpful, but as the disease progresses, patients will forget to use the devices, which may increase the risk of falling over them.
- Older persons easily become deconditioned and weak if not allowed to walk due to an intercurrent illness.
- Many of the medications given to such patients result in orthostatic hypotension or a drop in blood pressure when standing.
- Poor lighting and diminished visual ability contribute to the risk of falls and unsafe ambulation.

Possible Solutions to Ambulation Difficulties

- Many facilities now use scoop mattresses, which make it harder for patients to get up alone; but one cannot rely on equipment alone to prevent falls.
- In many facilities, personal alarm mechanisms are attached to the bed, chair, and person to alert staff when patients are trying to get up. Reminding patients or scolding them to call for help is not effective due to short-term memory loss.
- Frequent checks by staff can help to prevent falls, but clearly patients cannot be observed at arm's length 24 hours a day.
- During acute illnesses in hospitals, the use of family members or sitters is far superior to the use of restraints, which increase the risk for injury.

Fall Assessment and Prevention Protocols

Responsible long-term care facilities have fall assessment and prevention protocols in place. These involve an assessment of aspects intrinsic to the patient, including:

- Decreased muscle strength
- Gait disturbances including decreased arm swing
- Visual and other sensory deficits such as those seen in diabetics
- Medications that increase the risk of falls

Aspects extrinsic to the patient are also important and include:

- Low furniture
- Poor lighting
- Clutter
- Ill-fitting shoes
- Wet surfaces
- Lack of clearly visible hand rails on walls

Due to the high proportion of dementia patients in long-term care, such patients must be closely supervised and the environment constantly monitored for fall risks. The issue of fall risk must be openly discussed with families when a patient is admitted to a facility, as there are no solutions to guarantee that the patient will not fall.

Prudent staff will record a pattern of falling, including time of day, location, activity the patient was involved in, what happened before the fall, relationship to medications, medical conditions, and staffing patterns and organization. Review of this information may help to identify possible solutions for an individual patient.

CONTINENCE

One of the most significant challenges in dementia care is maintaining continence. In early stages, patients may wet or soil themselves because they cannot find the bathroom in time or undress quickly enough. In middle stages, they may not be able to recognize the toilet or recall how to use a toilet. In late stages, patients lose the ability to recognize the need to void or defecate.

Strategies to Increase Continence

- Make the bathroom visible; keep doors open and lights on.
- Use loose-fitting clothing that is easy for the patient to manipulate.
- Assist patients with hygiene after voiding, as the risk for developing a urinary tract infection is great.

- Males need routine prostate exams, as urinary retention due to an enlarged prostate can lead to a urinary tract infection.
- Staff must learn to recognize the signs that a patient needs to use the bathroom and then accompany the person. Such clues can include restlessness and tugging on clothing.
- The best strategy is to place the patient on a toileting schedule. This involves taking the patient to the bathroom every 2 hours. Asking the patient if he or she needs to use the bathroom will often result in a negative response. Rather than asking, simply hold out your arm and say, "Let's go for a walk."
- In late stages when patients no longer can interpret the signs of a full bladder or bowel, incontinence products are indicated. Staff should refer to them as "underwear" instead of diapers. Most adults will resist the attempts to change a diaper as they have no realization that they need one.

CONSTIPATION

Diminished activity and a diet that is low in fiber and fluids can result in constipation. As delineated in the behavior management chapter, Chapter 6, the first indication of constipation may be a change in behavior. A careful review of medications may reveal some that have constipation as a side effect, such as sedating medications. The first step in the process of addressing constipation is correct documentation of each bowel movement. Once it is confirmed, most facilities have a protocol to address the situation. Under no circumstances should patients be scolded for soiling themselves.

GIVING MEDICATIONS

The elderly take many medications and it can be a significant challenge to persuade the patient with dementia to accept them. Patients may argue that they don't need medications, that their doctor didn't order them, or they may simply refuse to open their mouths.

General Guidelines for Giving Medications

- The first strategy is to simply offer the medications—often the patient will take them.
- Most medications (except extended release) can be crushed and put into a soft food that the patient will enjoy, such as pudding or ice cream. Use this approach for patients who refuse medications.
- Lengthy arguments about medications usually serve to increase the resistance of the patient.
- To diminish the number of times a patient must be approached to take medications, review the list of prescribed medicines and eliminate unnecessary ones.
- Note that many medications are now formulated in liquids or quickly dissolving tablets.

VITAL SIGNS, BLOOD DRAWS, AND WOUND CARE

General Guidelines

- If a patient resists taking vital signs, it is best to have two people present—one to do the measurement and one to talk to and distract the patient.
- With blood draws also use two people. Secure the arm from which the sample is to be taken over the other arm. The second person can talk to the patient while the procedure is taking place.
- When a patient resists wound care, follow the rule of "Medicate before you manipulate." Pain medication can ease the discomfort of the procedure so it can be performed quickly and efficiently.
- Air splints will limit the mobility of an arm so that dressings and sutures will stay in place.
- When using IVs, wrap both extremities with cling bandages so the patient cannot see the tubes. Binders are also useful.

Chapter 6

MANAGING BEHAVIORAL PROBLEMS

Cynthia D. Steele

🔑 Key Points

- Importance of behavioral problems to dementia patient care
- Common behavioral issues
- Origins of behavioral complaints
- 5-D Strategy for resolving behavioral problems

While the defining hallmarks of dementia are impairments in cognition and function, it is often the case that problems in behavioral are more troubling to family and professional caregivers. At the start, it is important for the nurse to realize that the behavioral problems of the dementia patient can be managed. Keep these key principles in mind:

1. Management of behavioral problems is an important aspect of dementia care.
2. There are multiple possible causes and effective responses.
3. Trial and error are essential strategies.
4. A common language and definition of observable behavioral is essential to the process of assessment and management and must be used consistently by all staff.

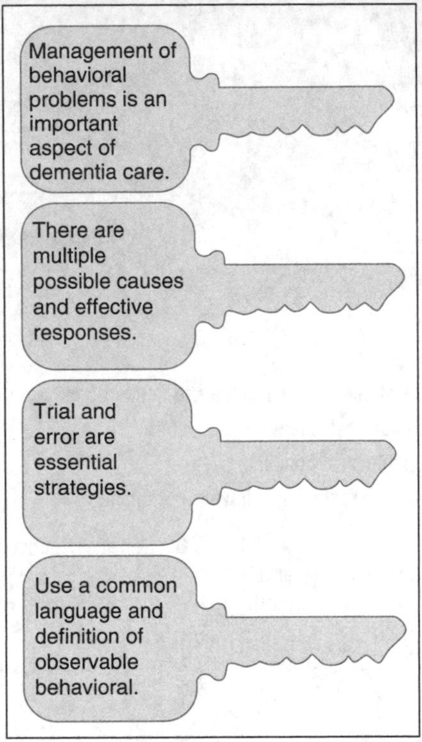

- Management of behavioral problems is an important aspect of dementia care.
- There are multiple possible causes and effective responses.
- Trial and error are essential strategies.
- Use a common language and definition of observable behavioral.

Figure 6-1   Keys to behavioral management.

SIGNIFICANCE OF BEHAVIORAL PROBLEMS IN DEMENTIA CARE

Behavioral problems are an essential focus of dementia care because they are:

- Common—over 90% of patients will have at least one behavioral problem.
- Burdensome—resulting in significant difficulties for caregivers, family, and professionals.
- Most often the reason patients are taken to a health care professional—whether to the emergency department, primary care, or other health care services.
- Frequent reasons for institutionalization.
- Reasons for discharge from community settings such as day care or home care.
- A factor in the increased cost of care.

MOST COMMON BEHAVIORAL COMPLAINTS

It is helpful for the nurse to understand the types of behavioral problems that are common in patients with dementia care. These problems are typically a result of how the brain is affected by the disease, rather than an unwillingness of the patient to cooperate or behave properly. Common complaints are listed here.

- Uncooperativeness
- Refusing to bathe
- Refusing medications
- Resisting care
- Attempting to leave a safe area
- Getting lost
- Screaming "Help me! Help me!"
- Combativeness, hitting, scratching, grabbing, spitting, slapping, kicking
- Pulling out tubes, IVs
- Getting out of bed unsafely

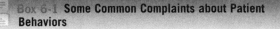

Box 6-1 Some Common Complaints about Patient Behaviors

- "She says she hasn't eaten in days and she just finished breakfast."
- "I tell him to get dressed and he just sits there."
- "He puts his clothes on inside out."
- "His manners are terrible."
- "I tell him to pick up his shirt and he looks and can't find it right in front of him."
- "She sits at the dining table and tries to eat her napkin."
- "I can't get her out of bed in the morning."
- "He says the medication is poison."
- "He is grabbing at the nursing aide's breasts."
- "Every weekend she refuses to dress and eat."

COMMON MYTHS AND REALITIES ABOUT BEHAVIORAL PROBLEMS

There are common myths and realities about behavioral problems in dementia patients.

MYTH: "Behavioral problems come out of nowhere."
REALITY: "There is always a trigger."

MYTH: "Behavioral problems cannot be predicted."
REALITY: "There is almost always a pattern to the behavioral outburst."

MYTH: "Behavioral problems are just deliberate acts of patients trying to be difficult."
REALITY: "Behavioral problems are the result of something in or around the patient."

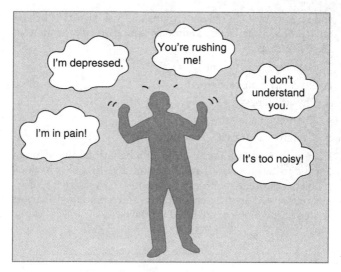

Figure 6-2   What is this patient trying to communicate?

MYTH: "Nothing can be done."
REALITY: "There is always an answer but trial and error are essential."

ORIGINS AND RISK FACTORS OF BEHAVIORAL PROBLEMS

Five Domains

There are five domains that are typically related to behavioral problems. Often more than one domain is involved. Careful and systematic review of the domains often leads to the identification of the issue triggering the behavioral. This allows the nurse to plan a rational approach for diminishing the frequency and severity of the problem. Origins and risk factors of behavioral problems are most commonly found in one or more of these five areas:

1. Cognitive impairment
2. Psychiatric problems
3. Physical illness
4. Environmental impact
5. Caregiver approach

Each of the risk factors can result in a behavioral that is problematic to caregivers. What follows are five lists of behavioral problems associated with each domain. The underlying problems are listed in the left column, and common behaviors related to the problem are listed on the right.

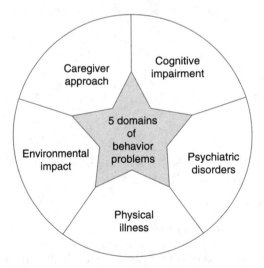

Figure 6-3   Domains of behavioral problems.

Domain 1: Cognitive Impairment (The 4 A's)

Underlying Problem	Common Behaviors
• Amnesia: Inability to form new memories	• After eating breakfast, the patient may say, "I haven't been fed in days!" • After a patient's husband leaves, the patient may say, "When is my husband coming to visit?"
• Aphasia: Inability to find words or understand them	• Telling a patient to get dressed and he or she just sits there with no reaction. • The patient says, "I want that!" and reaches for something, but can't identify what "that" is.
• Apraxia: Inability to perform learned motor movements	• The patient puts his or her clothes on inside out and buttons them incorrectly. • The patient appears to have terrible manners, picking up food with his or her hands and refusing to use a knife and fork.
• Agnosia: Inability to recognize objects and people	• The patient is told to put on his or her shirt and can't find it, even though the shirt is in plain view. • In the bathroom, the patient just stands there or may urinate in the sink and try to wash his or her hands in the toilet bowl. • The patient sits at the dining table and attempts to eat his or her napkin.

Domain 2: Psychiatric Disorders

Underlying Problem	Common Behaviors
• Depression	• Patient won't get out of bed in the morning.
	• Patient who used to enjoy activities will no longer participate.
	• Patient cries all the time but is not sad.
	• Patient wanders around in the middle of the night looking distraught.
• Delusions	• Patient won't take medication because he or she says it is poisoned.
	• Patient states another resident has stolen his or her belongings.
	• Patient won't go upstairs, believing that strangers are living there.
• Hallucinations	• Patient points under his or her bed, stating there is an animal or creature there.
	• Patient refuses to go into his or her room at night.
• Mania	• Patient makes sexual overtures to caregivers and touches them inappropriately.
	• Patient tells everyone they must leave because he is the king now.
	• Patient continually walks—even through the night, shows signs of irritability, speaks quickly and places his face too close to others.

Domain 3: Physical Illness

Underlying Problem	Common Behaviors
• Pain in hip after an unwitnessed fall	• Patient hits the aide when the aide touches his or her leg.
• Tooth decay	• Patient is losing weight and won't eat. He or she also pushes others away when they try to perform mouth care.
• Constipation	• Patient is eating less and guards the abdomen when he is showered.
• Urinary tract infection	• Patient states he or she has to go to the bathroom every 10 minutes and does not urinate.
	• The urine in patient's undergarments is dark and foul smelling.
	• Patient holds genital area and moans.
• Discomfort from sitting all day in the same position	• Patient tries to get up and walk unsafely.
• Delirium due to medication side effects	• Patient is too sleepy to eat much.

Domain 4: Environmental Impact

Underlying Problem	Common Behaviors
• Loud music in the dining room	• Patient won't stay in the dining room long enough to eat.
• Someone is screaming at another patient	• Patient tries to run away; pounds on the door trying to get out.
• Watching the evening news	• Patient calls 911 to tell authorities his or her spouse has been kidnapped.
• Temperature too hot	• Patient walks out of his or her room undressed.

Domain 5: Caregiver Approach

Underlying Problem	Common Behaviors
• Untrained weekend staff	• Every weekend, patient refuses to dress and eat.
	• "as needed, or prn" medications used when unfamiliar staff is on duty.
• Demanding, threatening staff	• Patient cries during meals when the staff states that if the patient doesn't immediately eat, they will take the food away.
• Giving multistage commands	• Patient completes one step of a task and then stops.
	• The aide asks the nurse to get medication for this uncooperative patient.
• Several aides attempt to hold the patient down for a bed bath	• The patient bites caregivers' arms and spits at them.

It is clear to see that there are many reasons why dementia patients are at high risk for behavioral problems. Their cognitive impairment, common psychiatric disorders, physical illness, environmental impact, and the caregiver approach may result in what caregivers define as problematic behavioral. There is, however, a systematic way of understanding the underlying triggers of problematic behavioral. Once such triggers are identified, a rational plan of care to address them can be devised.

THE 5-D STRATEGY

Prevention and Management of Behavioral Problems

The 5-D Strategy provides a systematic way to logically understand behavioral problems and provides a framework for planning to avoid these problems in the future. The following are the key elements of this strategy. For each behavioral observed:

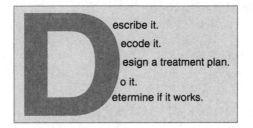

Figure 6-4   5-D Strategy.

1. Describe it.
2. Decode it.
3. Design a treatment plan.
4. Do it.
5. Determine if it works.

Here is how to follow each step of the 5-D Strategy.

Describe It

Helpful Descriptions

One of the most challenging parts of behavioral management is accurately and concisely describing the problematic behavioral. Helpful descriptions include only the facts and answer these questions:

- What did you see and hear?
- Where did it happen?
- When did it happen?
- What happened just before the behavioral was observed?
- During what activity or circumstances?
- With whom?
- How often does the behavioral occur?

Unhelpful Descriptions

Note that a poor description can make matters worse by confusing the situation and adding extraneous and unimportant detail. Avoid these types of statements in your descriptions:

• Vague statements: "She just went off on me."

• Judgmental statements: "He has always been nasty."

• Critical statements: "I know she is just trying to make my day worse."

Box 6-2 Helpful Descriptions

Example of a helpful description: Mrs. S was in the dining room with Mr. R. The TV was loud. Mr. R came up to her and just stood there staring at her. She stood up and hit him in the arm with a clenched fist.

Example of a description that is not helpful: Mrs. S and Mr. R got into it again today as always. She (Mrs. S) was her usual nasty self and went after Mr. R.

Decode It

To decode the behavioral problem, identify all the domains that could be contributing to the underlying problem. The domains are cognitive impairment, psychiatric problems, physical illness, environmental impact, and caregiver approach. Ask these types of questions to determine the domain.

Cognition

• How cognitively impaired is the patient?

• Is it possible the patient could have misinterpreted someone's actions?

• The nurse must directly test the cognitive abilities of the patient and determine if there has been a sudden change in cognitive impairment.

Psychiatric Disorders

- Has the patient developed a new psychiatric disorder, such as a delusion or depression?
- The nurse must interview the patient directly to determine if a new disorder is present.

Physical Illness

Remember! A change in behavioral is often the first sign of an emerging medical illness.

- Has the patient developed a new illness recently?
- Have new medications been prescribed?
- Are possible sources of pain leading to irritability?

You must directly examine the patient and review his or her medications. Notice if chronic conditions are stable or if a new medical condition has arisen. Examine the patient from head to toe by inspection and palpation; conduct a body audit.

Environmental Impact

- What was going on in the environment when the patient demonstrated the behavioral?
- Were there loud noises or disturbing programming on TV?
- Were there other upset patients in the area?

Caregiver Approach

- How did the caregiver react to a behavioral problem?
- Did the caregiver's reaction make the behavioral better or worse?
- Is the caregiver unfamiliar with the patient and his or her impairments?

Design a Treatment Plan

Design a plan based on the results of decoding and the identification of likely sources of the behavioral problem. A rational approach with concrete information about the incident can lead to a plan that will begin to deal with the problem. The clinical team should provide a definition of success. This gives the team confidence that if the plan does not work, there will be further attempts to solve the problem. If the problem continues to occur, revisit and revise the plan until an effective response is identified. Remember that trial and error are an expected part of the process.

Do It

Excellent behavioral management plans often fail due to the lack of consistent implementation. The plans must be written in simple language and provided to and explained to the persons who will implement them. This is most often the nursing assistant or care technician.

Monitoring the Plan

The success or failure of the plan must be reported at shift change between the aides in order to determine if the plan needs to be modified. Simple monitoring of outcomes can be accomplished by putting a sheet of graph paper in the nursing aide report book with blocks for each hour of the shift and a "+" or "−" indicating whether the behavioral occurred that hour or not.

Dealing with Irregular Shifts

A succinct plan is especially important for shifts that float on other units or only work occasionally. Weekend and agency staff must also work from the same plan.

Role of the Nurse Leader

Because the success of the plan often has to do with subtle issues such as how to greet and approach a patient, the effective nurse or team leader will want to demonstrate the correct approach and allow the staff to observe. The nursing leader who is not willing to engage the difficult patient will quickly lose credibility with the staff and they will be less likely to attempt the suggested plan. Since most behavioral problems occur during bathing, the effective leader must be willing to get wet along with the aide. Praise should be given for consistent attempts to implement the plan even if it fails.

Determine If It Works

Using the definition of success as defined by the clinical team, determine if the plan is reducing or eliminating the problem behavioral. Trial and error are expected. An emergency plan should also be devised, particularly when patients are aggressive. An example of an emergency plan is: "If the plan is implemented and the patient hits the staff two more times, the psychiatrist will be called and other measures considered."

Not only does the alternative plan apply a secondary approach to eliminating the behavioral, but it helps to prevent staff from getting demoralized and thinking that there never will be a solution to the problem. Demoralized staff members are more likely to retaliate against patients and eventually will either refuse to care for the problematic patient or quit.

In conclusion, the best way to deal with behavioral problems is to adjust your expectations to the abilities of the patient, recognize and treat physical and psychiatric disorders, moderate the environment to the patient's tolerance, and fine-tune the caregiver approach.

ILLUSTRATION OF THE 5-D STRATEGY

Problem Behavioral

The volume of the television in the dining room was high. Mrs. S was in the dining room with Mr. R. Mr. R approached Mrs. S and proceeded to stare at her. Mrs. S stood up and hit Mr. R in the arm with a clenched fist.

Describe the Behavioral

Mrs. S was in the dining room with Mr. R. The TV was loud. Mr. R came up to her and just stood there staring at her. She stood up and hit him in the arm with a clenched fist.

Decode the Behavioral

Mr. R's dementia had progressed to the point that he was no longer verbal and Mrs. S had developed a delusional disorder resulting in her belief that "all the men here will hurt me." A review of the caregiver's behavioral revealed that she shouted "Mrs. S, he won't hurt you, you are being mean to him. Stop it!" This made the patient even more frightened and threatened.

Design the Treatment

Identified triggers:

- Mrs. S was suffering from a delusion that all men were going to hurt her. Mr. R's presence frightened her.
- Mr. R was mute and could not converse with Mrs. S.
- The caregiver criticized Mrs. S, making her feel more threatened.

A meeting is held where the incident is discussed and triggers are identified. The following plan is made:

1. After both patients are evaluated for emerging physical illnesses and none found, Mrs. S will be seen by the psychiatrist to confirm that she has a delusional disorder needing treatment. If the treatment includes psychotropic medications, their side effects will be monitored.

2. Temporarily, Mrs. S will sit in a dining room in an area where she faces only women.

3. If a man approaches her, he will be redirected by staff.

4. The television will be turned off in the dining room to reduce confusing noise.

5. This plan will be written down and communicated to all staff including weekend and agency.

6. At a planned meeting next week, the supervising nurse will report on the progress of the plan and necessary changes will be made.

7. The supervising nurse will demonstrate behaviors to redirect male patients away from Mrs. S and also will demonstrate how to provide reassurance to Mrs. S that she will be safe.

8. If an approaching male patient cannot be moved, Mrs. S will be escorted from the area.

9. The plan is successful if Mrs. S's aggressive behavioral in the dining room is reduced by 50% in the first week.

Do It

The plan is provided to all team members, including weekend staff. The plan is explained to all appropriate staff members with leaders watching that the plan is implemented.

Determine If It Works

After one week, the clinical staff reviews the plan. Mrs. S's aggressive behavioral was reduced by 90% in the dining room. Although one incident did occur, it was due to poor communication between temporary staff persons who were working in the dining room.

MANAGING AGGRESSIVE BEHAVIORAL

Some behaviors are easy to ignore and others require analysis and resolution. Aggressive behavioral can cause situations that upset both staff and patients.

General Information

Aggressive behavioral has been defined as:

> Any behavioral that threatens or causes harm to self, others, or objects. Aggressive behaviors include kicking, hitting, biting, grabbing, spitting, slapping and other forceful actions.

The significance of aggressive behavioral lies in the fact that once a patient is described as aggressive, the staff may avoid the person. Some staff may even refuse to care for these patients.

- Aggressive behaviors most commonly occur during direct personal care. Nursing aides and family members are greatly impacted.
- It is a salient reason for a facility or service to discharge a patient.
- It may certainly be linked to aides choosing to change jobs if they feel there is no answer or way to avoid the behavioral.

Cues and Micro-Cues

At times it may be obvious that a patient is escalating toward an aggressive episode. Indicators of escalation include:

- Tension in muscles
- Restlessness, pacing about
- Furrowed brow, angry-appearing face
- Loud voice, whether making threats or not

See Table 6-1 for appropriate responses to escalating aggression.

Remember that it is most always easier to remove those at risk from an area where a patient is escalating rather than trying to remove the upset patient. When everyone on the clinical team is trained in response to aggression, they can act in a coordinated fashion and often avoid any injury or the need to transfer the patient.

Tips to Reduce Aggression

- Reduce noise.
- Do not call out the cavalry.
- Reduce lighting.

Table 6-1   Cycle of Escalation and Appropriate Response

Patient	Staff Response
Anxious, fretful	Reassure, use gentle touch.
Angry	Listen but do not touch, give space.
Hostile	Start making a plan of action, survey the environment for those at risk.
Aggressive	Allow to de-escalate (calm down) if possible. If not, use nonoffensive physical control to prevent harm to the patient and those around the patient.

- Eliminate anything the patient perceives as a threat, such as a loud peer.
- Avoid charging a patient, which can often result in an exaggerated reaction.
- Have only one person talk to the patient.

Try to avoid the use of prn, or as needed, sedating medications. Although these medications usually provide sedation, they often make a patient even more confused and do not solve the problem.

The nurse and aides may wish to attend a class to learn a "safe hold" or "secure hold." This is a method of holding a patient so the individual cannot hurt others or himself or herself. It allows the patient to be moved to a safe area.

MANAGING SEXUAL BEHAVIORS

Careful Analysis Is Required

Health care staff may have a great deal of anxiety about potential sexual behaviors exhibited by a demented patient. Before labeling a behavioral as sexual in nature, a careful analysis is necessary. For example, a male patient who has apraxia may emerge from the bathroom with his genitals exposed, due to the limitations of apraxia, which prevent him from zipping his pants.

It is important to understand that all people seek human contact and companionship. In a nursing home or assisted living facility this can be problematic. For example, a patient with dementia may misidentify another as his or her spouse, or a patient may attempt to engage in intimate physical behavioral with someone too impaired to give consent.

Patient Misinterpretations

It is not uncommon for patients to misinterpret the actions of staff as sexually inviting. This can happen when staff refer to patients as "honey" or "sweetheart" and hug the patients. Staff members must be vigilant about their approach to patients. If a female member of the staff leans over a patient who is in a wheelchair, she may inadvertently place her breasts in the face of the patient, who may then grope the staff member. Rather than labeling the patient a sexual deviant, it is better to rethink the situation and approach the patient from the side.

Appropriate Responses

It is always appropriate to say to a patient, "Stop. I am your nursing assistant, that is not appropriate behavioral." In some instances, usually with sexually aggressive males, hormonal treatments can be considered.

Chapter 7

DESIGNING ACTIVITIES

Cynthia D. Steele and Stephen Vozzella ACC, BA

Key Points

- Benefits of activities for patients with dementia
- Assessing a patient's interests
- How to plan, lead, and evaluate activities
- Activities appropriate to all stages of dementia

People with dementia benefit from engaging in activities.[1] Because they are a vital part of life, activities should be incorporated into every health care setting—both in the hospital and in chronic care environments, such as day care centers, nursing homes, and home care. Anyone can initiate an activity with a patient and it need not be an expensive or time-consuming endeavor.

THE BENEFITS OF ACTIVITIES

Activities are an important part of a person's day, just as important as medicine, therapy, and rest. For a person with dementia, activities need to be provided just like a prescription. Activities are a particularly important part of the dementia patient's day, because the patient may:

- Have forgotten WHAT activities he or she enjoyed
- Forget HOW TO DO activities he or she enjoyed
- Be unable TO PLAN activities himself or herself

Specifically, activities provide the following benefits for people with dementia:

- Relaxation
- Stress relief
- Success at accomplishment[2]
- Purposefulness
- Creative outlets
- Companionship (if desired)
- Spirituality
- Fitness

ASSESSING A DEMENTIA PATIENT'S ACTIVITY NEEDS

The assessment of each patient is critical to identifying what the person previously enjoyed and the person's current capabilities. Activities must be individualized to be successful. Information about an individual's past can provide bridges to helping him or her now.

How to Conduct an Assessment

1. Interview Persons Who Know the Patient

- Talk to family members who have lived with the person for extended periods.
- Talk to the patient.
- If no family members are available, talk to a friend who has known the patient for a long time.

2. Learn about the Patient's Personal History

- BIRTHPLACE. People with dementia typically identify with their hometown.
- PLACES WHERE THEY HAVE LIVED. People with dementia tend to remember the places they lived in their teens and 20s.
- FAMILY MEMBERS AND FRIENDS. People with dementia may recall spouse, parents' names, children's names, and

grandchildren (but do not expect them to remember how many or all their names).

- OCCUPATION. People with dementia may respond to a past role, especially one that encompassed a large part of their years or took place in their earlier years.
- LANGUAGE. People with dementia tend to speak the language they first learned.
- EDUCATION. Find out the names of schools the patient attended and studies of interest; the patient may respond to a school song or mascot.
- FOODS. Find out if the person has food allergies and identify his or her favorite foods, as this may be all he or she eats.
- TYPICAL DAY. Determine how the person prefers to spend the day—sleeping, staying up late, napping, busy?
- MAJOR EVENTS. Find out what significant events occurred in the patient's life; this may give you something to talk about.
- VISION. Identify the type of visual-related assistance the person will need to participate in an activity.
- HEARING. Identify the type of hearing-related assistance the person will need to participate in an activity.
- DOMINANT HAND. Determine which hand the person uses for writing and which is the stronger hand; this helps to identify if the person needs physical assistance to participate in activities.

3. Identify Activities of Interest

People with dementia often demonstrate an interest in a surprising number and variety of activities. Use the following list of possible activities to identify those suitable for a particular patient. See Box 7-1, "Coding Interests."

- Books
- Current events
- Newspapers
- Crocheting
- Sewing
- Knitting
- Reminiscing
- Socializing
- Spirituality
- Magazines

- Collecting
- TV
- Radio
- Movies
- Cats
- Dogs
- Other pets
- Shopping
- Bingo
- Cards
- Board games
- Crosswords
- Jigsaws
- Baking
- Cooking
- Chores
- Drawing
- Flower arranging
- Painting
- Photography
- Other arts
- Writing
- Computers
- Gardening
- Houseplants
- Outings
- Travel
- Clubs
- Politics
- Organizations
- Volunteering
- Humor
- Intergenerational
- Concerts
- Opera
- Plays
- Listening to music
- Bowling
- Dancing
- Exercising
- Golf
- Sports fan
- Swimming
- Tennis
- Other sports
- Walking
- Outdoors
- General other

4. Determine Current Abilities for Participation

- Independent. Can start activities on own.
- Dependent. Needs help to do activities.
- Active observer. Observes activities, comments, shows expression.
- Passive observer. Observes part of the time, no verbal comments or nonverbal expression.

> **Box 7-1 Coding Interests**
>
> It is important to note whether or not the patient has an interest in the areas listed, and specifically note what the interest is. For example, if the person says she likes cards, then find out exactly what kind of cards she likes to play. It is also important to note the interest even if the person doesn't do the activity anymore.
>
> Example:
>
> • Cards P: Used to enjoy solitaire in the past.
> • Tennis N: Never been an interest.
> • Music C: Currently enjoys listening to Frank Sinatra.
>
> *Key: C, current interest; P, past interest; N, never been an interest.*

* Passive unaware. Is unaware when activity is occurring.
* Refuses. Does not want to participate in anything.

5. **Review Assessment and Make a Plan**
   * What activities does the person like?
   * How do the activities need to be adapted to the person's current abilities?
   * What help does the person need to participate?
   * In assisted living or long-term care, an interdisciplinary plan for the whole day should be created. The plan should include sleep times, favorite activities, key friends and family members, toileting needs, bathing needs, dressing needs, toileting schedules, and meal needs. In the hospital, spontaneous or drop-off activities may suffice.

SELECTING ACTIVITIES

In the hospital environment, it does not take a large staff or expensive supplies to provide activities to patients with dementia.

Building pleasure into routine activities, such as sitting and talking with a patient about a picture on the wall or having coffee, is helpful. Drop-off activities, such as placing an object or magazine in the person's lap or hands, are effective ways to distract the patient from crawling out of bed or pulling out tubes.

In the chronic care environment, both simple and more extensive activities are appropriate. An example of a simple activity is to provide a used wallet or purse so the patient has something to hold and something for storing small items. An extensive activity might involve taking patients on an outing. In long-term care facilities, a nurse or designated activity staff should develop a plan for each person.

Box 7-2 Getting Patients to Participate to an Activity

Some patients with dementia will refuse to participate in activities when asked. Sometimes the patient does not understand the question, so he or she says "no." The best approach is to pose your communication as a clear and simple statement rather than a question.

SAY: "Let's go for a walk." or "Let's have some fun."

DON'T SAY: "Would you like to go for a walk?" or "Do you want to go to a fun activity?"

SIX CATEGORIES OF ACTIVITIES

Activities that are appropriate for people with dementia can be organized into six categories: intellectual, spiritual, physical, social, creative, and diversional. The ideal activity plan enables the patient to partake in activities from as many categories as possible.

Intellectual

- Reading aloud
- Biographies

- Books on tape
- Slide shows
- Name that tune
- Current events
- Trivia

Spiritual

- Radio mass
- Prayer books
- Clergy visits
- Bible on tape
- Study of religious texts
- Spiritual songs or hymns on tapes

Physical

- Chair exercise
- Dancing—standing or in a chair
- Basketball
- Swimming
- Golf—putting golf balls
- Balloon ball
- Walking

Social

- Tea party
- Lemonade social
- Milkshake party
- Happy hour—alcohol-free drinks
- Discussion groups
- Reminisce
- Live entertainment
- Meet with friends

Creative

- Paint by numbers
- Ceramics
- Cooking
- Flower arranging
- Baking
- Collages

Diversional

- Trips to places of interest
- Sing-along
- Bingo
- Sensory stimulation
- Fish tanks
- Plants
- Scenery
- Birds
- Music

PLANNING AN ACTIVITY

Planning ahead is the best way to ensure that an activity is successful. If the activities staff or nurse has assessed the person's interests, the next step is to find resources to plan activities that pertain to the patient's interests and abilities.

Resources for Activity Planning

- Activity assessment
- Internet
- Library
- Second-hand stores
- Basement/attic

Box 7-3 How to Adapt an Activity (Chronic Care Environment)

There are many creative ways to adapt activities to a person's abilities, as in this example for a person who likes fishing. In the hospital, you might give the patient a magazine about fishing.

- Early stages—Take the patient to a local fishing area: need help baiting hook.
- Middle stages—Watch fishing show and discuss: fish indoors using a magnet on pole and paper fish that have paper clips on them that attract the magnet.
- Late stages—Look at photos of fishing, touch the fishing rod, go on a scenic drive that includes stopping at a fishing hole.

Important note: It is always beneficial to keep the activity as simple as possible. Always consider how to break the activity into steps and do one thing at a time.

Box 7-4 How to Adapt an Activity (Hospital Environment)

To adapt an activity to a hospital setting, simplify and scale it down to the person's ability level and to the limited space and resources of the environment. Here is an example for a person who likes to play the piano.

- Early stages—Bring the patient a portable keyboard and place it on his or her lap so it can be played in bed or while sitting in a chair.
- Middle stages—Discuss favorite songs to play on the piano, discuss famous piano players, play music trivia, reminisce how the person learned to play. For example, say "How many of you enjoyed Frank Sinatra?" or "What was your favorite song?"
- Late stages—Listen to piano pieces, look at photos of famous piano players, and look at photos of different styles of pianos.

Important note: It is always beneficial to keep the activity as simple as possible. Always consider how to break the activity into steps and do one thing at a time.

- Newspaper
- Magazines

Planning an Activity

- Plan ahead.
- Plan using the person's interests.
- Plan for half-hour increments.
- Have a backup plan, such as a balloon, short story, travel pictures, or something that always catches the patient's attention.
- Adapt a favorite activity.

LEADING AN ACTIVITY

Types of Activities Nurses Can Lead

- Group—activity with 2 or more people
- Individual—activity with 1 person
- Drop-off—activity you give to the person and then back away
- Spontaneous—an unplanned activity that emerges from looking around the room or comes as a great idea, such as discussing a family photo, singing a song on the radio, or reading a story in a magazine
- Environment—fish tanks, paintings, plants, music, etc.

Leading Group Activities

Before You Start

- Have supplies ready to start.
- Choose a quiet place to meet, turn off televisions or radios, and reduce any outside noise. (*Individual activity—pick a place that is familiar to the person or a place with familiar pictures or objects.*)
- Do not use a table unless you need it, remove the patient from the area. (*In a group setting—sit people in a circle or semicircle.*)
- Have your back-up plan ready—have a balloon, short story, travel pictures, or something you know never fails.

- Make sure room temperature is comfortable; it should probably be on the warm side.
- In a group setting—do not sit people who do not get along near one another.
- Remove bright light or glare.
- Plan to have hearing-impaired persons sit near the leader or use adaptive devices, such as an amplifier.

While You Are Leading
- Be patient.
- Be energetic.
- Welcome the person or persons depending on what type of group it is.
- Introduce yourself.
- Give each person a chance to introduce him or herself. Introduce patients if they are not able to.
- Introduce the activity.
- Give each person a chance to participate.
- Break the activity into as many steps as possible and give praise for each step completed.
- Speak slowly and clearly.
- Be aware of body language—nonverbal language is as important as words.
- Conclude the activity with a question—for example, "Would you do this again?" or "Did you like this activity?"
- Observe the process—pay attention to how persons participate and note it afterwards. Use this information for evaluation to see if you will need to modify it if it is repeated.
- Thank each person for attending.

After the Activity Is Over
In chronic care settings, documentation is very important. This is accomplished by noting the level of the patient's participation, the amount of cueing required, and his or her apparent enjoyment of the activity. The codes listed in Box 7-5 allow for thoughtful but expedient documentation.

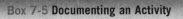

Box 7-5 Documenting an Activity

Copper Ridge Activity Index[3]

Participation:

- I = Independent participation, participant initiates the activity
- D = Participates with assist
- AO = Active Observer, provides comments, facial expressions
- PO = Passive Observer
- PU = Passive Unaware
- R = Refused

Cueing:

- Min = Minimum amounts of cueing needed for the person to participate, or 0–33% of your time was required.
- Mod = Moderate amounts of cueing needed for the person to participate, or 34–66% of your time was required.
- Max = Maximum amounts of cueing needed for the person to participate, or 67–100% of your time was required.

Apparent enjoyment rating:

- 1 = Dislikes the activity
- 2 = No response, flat affect
- 3 = Minimum enjoyment
- 4 = Moderate enjoyment
- 5 = Maximum enjoyment

HOW TO EVALUATE AN ACTIVITY

Evaluating an activity provides the nurse with important feedback for selecting successful activities in the future. Activities may be evaluated in terms of the leader's preparation and carry-through as well as the patient's participation and enjoyment. The forms in Figures 7-1 and 7-2 are useful for evaluating group and individual activities.

Activity _____

Activity led by _____

	Yes	No	N/A	Comments
Pre-planning of activity program is evident. Goal in place				
Circular seating arrangement				
Group size is appropriate for what is planned				
Attempt is made to involve each person in the group				
Program is success-oriented				
Tone and volume of leader enhances participation				
Program encourages independence				
Area is large enough				
Program is free from interruptions				
Group participants show interest in activity				
Program modifications are made to accommodate special needs of participants				
Participants are redirected by staff, appropriate interventions are used				

Figure 7-1   Evaluating group activity form.

Activity   _____

Activity led by _____

	Yes	No	N/A	Comments
Pre-planning of activity program is evident. Goal in place				
Program is success-oriented				
Tone and volume of leader enhances participation				
Program encourages independence				
Area is large enough				
Program is free from interruptions				
Participant shows interest in activity				
Program modifications are made to accommodate special needs of participant				
Participant is redirected by activity leader, appropriate interventions are used				

Figure 7-2   How to evaluate an individual activity.

ACTIVITIES THAT ARE SUCCESSFUL FOR EARLY, MIDDLE, AND LATE STAGES OF DEMENTIA

High-Functioning Activities

- Exercise—standing optional
- Water aerobics

- Painting class
- Glaze ceramics
- Museum trips
- Crossword puzzles
- Discuss recent newspaper articles
- Bingo
- Shopping trips
- Reading to children
- Jigsaw puzzles
- Bible study
- Computer games
- Card games
- Golfing

Moderate-Functioning Activities

- Water colors
- Dull-coat ceramics
- Reminisce historic events
- Baking and cooking simple recipes
- Walking groups
- Putting golf balls
- Reciting prayers
- Music trivia (give them half the answer)
- Trips to restaurants
- Watering flowers
- Folding clothes, papers, etc.
- Car wash

Low-Functioning Activities

These activities are appropriate for persons who are bed bound.
- Hand massages
- Smelling spices

- Looking at pictures from the person's past
- Listening to music
- Music sing-a-longs
- Making Jell-O, applesauce, pudding
- Ball toss, balloon toss
- Chair dancing
- Short walks
- Prayer readings, musical hymns

ACTIVITIES FOR PEOPLE WITH BEHAVIOR PROBLEMS

There are times when people with dementia exhibit behavior problems. The activity assessment may help the nurse or activities staff plan activities that are specific to a person's behavior issue. The following suggested activities help address different behavior problems. Try several different approaches until you find one that is successful for the patient.

Wandering

- Give magazine or book for browsing
- CD and headphones to provide stimulation
- Massage
- Stationary bike
- Take person for a walk

Yelling

- Headphones for music
- Stuffed animal or doll for comfort
- Massage
- Volunteer for one-on-one activity

Repetitive Movement—Pulling Bandages, Tubes, Etc.

- Magazines
- Stuffed animals or dolls
- Hand-held puzzles
- Ball
- Balloon

Anxiety

Familiar activities can help.
- Dancing
- Shredding cheese
- Walking
- Baseball toss
- Painting
- Pet therapy
- Reminisce
- Picture trivia
- Walking
- Picture cards

REFERENCES

1. Bowlby C. *Therapeutic Activities with Persons Disabled by Alzheimer disease and Related Disorders*. Gaithersburg, MD: Aspen; 1993.
2. Zgola JM. *Care That Works: A Relationship Approach to Persons with Dementia*. Baltimore: John Hopkins University Press; 1999.
3. Politis AM, Vozzella S, Mayer LS, Onyike CU, Baker AS, Lyketsos CG. A randomized, controlled, clinical trial of activity therapy for apathy in patients with dementia residing in long-term care. *Int J Geriatr Psychiatry*. 19:1087-1094; 2004.

Chapter 8

HELPING FAMILIES

Cynthia D. Steele

🔑 Key Points

- The special challenges of the primary caregiver
- Gathering information from caregivers
- Educating and guiding caregivers
- Identifying community resources
- Providing emotional support

Family members play a crucial role in the well-being of their loved one with dementia. Regardless of whether a patient with dementia resides in a residential care facility or is in the hospital for a brief stay, family members are a main source of patient information and supplemental patient care. It is important that nurses understand the profound impact that dementia has on caregivers and on the family in general. The effective nurse can provide essential information and support to the caregiver of a patient with dementia.

CAREGIVERS OF DEMENTIA PATIENTS

Primary Caregivers

Most of the work in caring for persons with dementia is accomplished through caregivers. Who are they?

- Most are women, wives, daughters, and daughters-in-law.
- Many reduce or leave work to provide care.

• Most care is provided by this private, unpaid resource rather than paid help.

There is usually a "primary caregiver" who performs the majority of care, and thus experiences the burdens that are associated with constant care. There are no generic caregivers; each person faces the challenges of caring in his or her own characteristic way that must be understood.

Special Challenges

Since most dementia has a gradual onset, many caregivers do not recognize there is a significant problem with a family member until a crisis occurs. The person with dementia may get lost in familiar territory or leave a pot on the stove to burn. The individual may become disoriented and upset when taken away from his or her usual routine.

Hospitalization further stresses the demented patient due to constant noise, unfamiliar people, sedating medications, and disruptions in homeostasis from the illness itself and from anesthesia. Many families become convinced that "the surgery caused the dementia" because it was only in the post-op setting

---

Box 8-1 Stresses That May Amplify Dementia Impairments

• Changes in routine
• Loss of a caregiver
• Moving to a hospital or full-time care facility
• Dealing with strangers
• Hospital environment
• Sedating medications
• Illness
• Anesthesia

that the dementia became apparent. It is not uncommon for families to recognize cognitive impairments when a spouse who has been caring for the demented individual dies or is removed from the home due to sickness.

GATHERING INFORMATION FROM CAREGIVERS

Understanding the Caregiver

In order to provide the best possible care for a patient and his or her caregiver, the nurse must first identify three aspects of the family circumstances (see Figure 8-1):

1. Who is the primary caregiver? It is important to identify the primary caregiver, as he or she may not be the person who is admitting the patient for care. For example, an adult child may be admitting a patient for care, but an elderly spouse might be the primary caregiver.

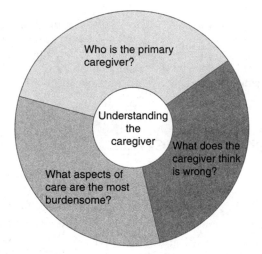

Figure 8-1   Understanding the caregiver.

2. What does the caregiver think is wrong with the patient's ability to function? Find out how much the caregiver understands about the patient's impairments.
3. What aspects of care are the most burdensome for the caregiver? This can help the nurse provide assistance and appropriate resources to the caregiver.

Interviewing Caregivers

Crucial information can be gleaned by interviewing caregivers. Not only can the nurse learn about the patient, but an interview provides an opportunity to see what type of assistance the family needs. It is essential to interview caregivers alone and away from the patient. Caregivers may not be fully forthcoming about the struggles they are experiencing in front of the patient, in an effort to protect the patient's dignity. In addition, if the person with dementia is present during an interview, the discussion about impairments may start arguments. Patients with dementia will often deny anything is wrong and accuse the caregiver of complaining.

Begin by asking the caregiver what he or she thinks is wrong with the patient. This will allow the nurse to identify and correct misinformation and myths. It is common for caregivers who are not educated about dementia to state, "He just isn't trying hard enough" or "She is just trying to make my life difficult."

ASSISTING CAREGIVERS

Consider these four basic goals when assisting caregivers:

1. Educate them about dementia.
2. Guide them in making decisions about the patient.
3. Identify community resources that can assist caregivers.
4. Provide emotional support to caregivers.

Educating Caregivers

Guidelines

During the process of educating caregivers, these simple guidelines can serve to improve communication and understanding:

- Use simple language.
- Utilize drawings of the brain.
- Reinforce, restate so they can understand, then repeat.
- Refer to the guidelines in the Appendix and provide these to the family.

Start with the Brain

A useful starting point when speaking with a caregiver is to show a simple drawing of the brain and explain the brain's normal functions. Laminated pictures of the lobes of the brain can be purchased at medical book stores or simple drawings can be found through other resources.

> **Box 8-2 Start with the Brain**
>
> Speak to caregivers about the brain. Because impairments are linked to the part of the brain that is damaged, it allows the caregiver to attribute impairments to failure of a brain region, rather than a willful act of stubbornness on the part of the patient.

Use simple language to explain dementia. Avoid words like "syndrome," as most will not understand it and may be reluctant to ask for clarification. It is often helpful to use a metaphor that is commonly understood, as explained in Box 8-3.

Box 8-3 How to Explain Dementia

When explaining dementia to caregivers, it is helpful to use a metaphor. One metaphor is to say that dementia is like the flu. The flu has well-recognized symptoms, such as aches, pains, and coughing. But the flu has many causes, such as Bangkok flu, Hong Kong flu, and so on. Similarly, dementia has symptoms, including memory loss, difficulty with language, recognizing the world, and performing functional tasks. But dementia also has many causes, including Alzheimer disease, stroke, inflammation of the brain, and others.

Discuss Specific Types of Dementia

If the diagnosis of the type of dementia has been made, it is useful to review the characteristic symptoms of that specific type and ask if the caregiver has noticed these symptoms.

Arrange a Family Care Team

Convening a family meeting to discuss the diagnosis and prognosis is often a very effective way to get members organized as a care team. It is not unusual for the social façade of the patient to remain intact even if the patient is very functionally impaired. Thus family members who do not live with or see the patient often may doubt the extent of the impairment.

Family meetings help to enlist others to assist the primary caregiver in providing help such as respite care. Common

Box 8-4 Educational Resources for Families

- ADEAR Center: www.nia.nih.gov/alzheimers
- Alzheimer Association: www.alz.org
- Family guidelines given in the Appendix

problems in engaging the family in care are (1) parents are reluctant to "burden" their children and (2) children do not know what course of action to take. Be sure to provide educational resources to the family.

Educate for the Appropriate Stage of Illness

Due to the progressive course of most dementing illnesses, caregiver and family education will focus on different issues at different stages of the disease. Table 8-1 presents a general guide to appropriate topics for early, middle, and late-stage illness.

Table 8-1   Topics to Discuss by Stage of Illness

Early-Stage Issues	Middle-Stage Issues	Late-Stage Issues
• Understanding the relative's illness	• Understanding and coping with behavior problems	• Possible placement in a nursing facility
• Treatment options, if any	• Driving	• Implementing decisions about end-of-life care
• Whether the patient should be told the diagnosis	• Handling money	• Assuring all family members are in agreement with the plan
• Whether it is safe to leave the patient alone	• Patient safety	
• Establishing a living will; identifying substitute decision-maker	• Adapting activities to keep the patient stimulated	
• Mobilizing the family to help as a care team	• Finding community resources	
	• Maintaining caregivers' emotional and physical well-being	
	• Finding respite care	
	• Assuring patient safety	
	• Making decisions about tube feeding, invasive diagnostic tests, trips to the hospital, innovation of hospice care	

Providing Instructions

When providing instructions about care, such as discharge instructions or how to take medications, be sure to explain all instructions to the caregiver and not just the patient alone. Although the patient may pay attention, he or she will not be able to remember the instructions, even if they are written down. Such documents must be given to and explained to the caregiver.

Providing Guidance to Caregivers

Delegating Responsibilities

Many decisions made by the person with dementia must be delegated to another. This can be a painful challenge for the caregiver if the patient does not recognize that his or her judgment is impaired. Relinquishing responsibilities is difficult for many persons with dementia. Key decisions that must be made include whether the person with dementia should:

- Handle money
- Continue to pay bills
- Continue to drive
- Make health care decisions alone
- Travel about unsupervised

Providing a Sense of Control

Obviously, if the patient has already made errors in handling money, such as forgetting to pay bills or losing documentation, these responsibilities should be taken over by someone trusted by the patient. This can be accomplished in a non-confrontational way by sitting with the patient and discussing the bill, then allowing the assisting person to write a check and the demented person to sign. This allows the patient to feel a sense of control. If bills and important documents are misplaced or lost, having these items sent to the address of the family member in charge can avoid confrontation.

Seek Legal Guidance

As early as possible in the illness, a surrogate decision-maker should be designated by the ill person if he or she still has the judgment to assign a trusted and responsible person. Lawyers who specialize in the management of the elderly can be of great help in advising the family as to whether the patient can still manage his or her affairs. The lawyer will often work along with the physician in making decisions about competency.

Living Wills

Elder attorneys are also helpful in drawing up a living will. This document includes decisions about what type of care the person with dementia wants and does not want. It is ideal if the ill person has input to the living will, but often the individual's judgment is too impaired to make such decisions. In such cases, which vary according to state law, surrogates make decisions in the best interest of the ill person with their best guess of what the person would have wanted. Living wills address issues such as:

* Feeding tubes
* Resuscitation
* Invasive medical testing
* Other medical interventions at the end of life

Guidance on Patient Driving

The nurse can greatly assist families in their decision-making process by making recommendations. For example, the nurse can recommend that the person with dementia should no longer drive. This can prevent the family from arguing about it. In some cases, a written prescription prohibiting driving is useful. Offices on Aging can often identify a local agency that can evaluate the ability to drive.

In the short term, the best driving test is to have a family member get in the car and observe the patient's ability. Another strategy is to ask the family member, "Would you allow your child to drive with this person?" Since driving requires simultaneously paying attention to multiple stimuli, dementia places the individual at great risk when driving. The goal here is to continue to allow the patient to get out of the house or facility, but to do so safely.

> **Box 8-5 What Are Your State's Driving Laws?**
>
> Some states, but not all, require that once a diagnosis of dementia is made, the patient must come in to the motor vehicle administration for an evaluation. Encourage caregivers to find out about the relevant driving laws in their state.

Identification Bracelets

Upon learning that a loved one suffers from dementia, it is important that families are proactive rather than reactive. For example, it is proactive to put identification on the patient before he or she wanders out. Instead, many families will say, "If she wanders out, then I'll put identification on her." Alternatives for persons who resist wearing a Medic Alert identification bracelet include:

- Giving a watch or attractive bracelet engraved with identification information as a gift
- Providing a baseball cap with the individual's name to identify the person in a crowd

Securing Important Documents

Memory-impaired patients frequently lose their wallets and other identification. It is wise to make copies of important information, such as Medicare cards, and give the copies to the patient. The caregiver can then keep the originals secure. See "Taking Inventory," Family Guidelines #15 in the Appendix.

Safety at Home

It is often useful to enlist the services of an occupational therapist to help determine if the patient is safe at home and specifically what tasks he or she can continue to do and which are too risky. It is best to have the therapist come to the home and observe the patient performing such tasks as cooking, calling for help in an emergency, and counting money. The occupational therapy evaluations conducted in a hospital are useful but not a perfect approximation of how a person functions in his or her familiar home environment. In some cases, it is possible for the patient to remain at home safely if preventative measures are taken. For example, if the person forgets to turn off the burners on the stove, a family member should disable the stove and have meals delivered or prepared by the family.

Identifying Resources

A variety of community resources can assist the family in the care of the dementia patient. Some resources that provide assistance to caregivers are listed in Table 8-2.

The majority of services that will be helpful are not paid for by health insurance, such as Medicare, and must be paid by the family directly. Some resources such as adult day care have sliding-scale fees. The expense of obtaining services must always be considered.

Table 8-2   Types of Community Resources

Type of Resource	What It Provides
Adult day care center	Activity, supervision, and respite
Assisted living facility	Housing and supervision
Nursing home	Medical supervision and housing
Meals on Wheels	Home-delivered meals
Medical alert bracelet	Identification of the patient
Home health care aide	Assistance in basic hygiene
Homemaker services	Assistance in cleaning, laundry, shopping, meal preparation
Department of Aging	Information and referral to resources in your area
Geriatric psychiatrist	Assistance with difficult behavior

Emotional Support for the Caregiver

Sharing Responsibilities

Social isolation, fatigue, and discouragement are common consequences of providing care to someone with dementia over the many years of illness. The first step in addressing this impact is to use the family meeting to rally support for the patient and caregiver. It is common for those in the family who are not involved with care to underestimate the burden experienced by the primary caregiver.

A family meeting provides an opportunity for the health care professional to review the diagnosis and impact of the illness and to make direct requests to divide up responsibilities. Since there is much to do, from personal care to paying bills for the person who is ill, responsibilities can be assigned to those in the family who feel comfortable with particular tasks. Family members who live out of town might be asked to contribute financially to hire someone to clean the house or take the person for a walk.

Providing Respite for the Caregiver

It is essential to sustain the caregiver's means of emotional support. Offers to stay with the patient while the caregiver goes to religious services or to lunch with friends are very important. It is not uncommon for the primary caregiver to neglect his or her own physical health in the process of caring for the person with dementia. Both the health care professional and the family should know what health problems the primary caregiver has and how these problems are being addressed. The caregiver must sustain his or her health through the many years of effort required to care for a loved one with dementia.

Many caregivers, especially women, are reluctant to make direct requests for help. The health care professional can assist in the process by coaching the caregiver to ask for specific time-limited assistance. A request as simple as, "Could you take John for a walk on Tuesdays?" can be very helpful for the patient, caregiver, and helper who is not sure what to do. Again, using the professional's recommendation is often useful, as with "The doctor says it is good for me to go to my exercise class weekly to be able to continue to care for John."

Mental Health Care

There is a perception that all caregivers become seriously depressed during the course of caregiving. Certainly that is true for some, but it is likely that most become distressed and demoralized by the seemingly endless nature of the illness. When appropriate, some caregivers will greatly benefit from having their own mental health care. Sources of such care can be sought from social workers, psychiatrists, and psychologists.

Support groups often conducted through the Office on Aging or the Alzheimer Association are often recommended as sources of support. It is important to know that this kind of support is generally most beneficial for those caregivers doing fairly well. During sessions, caregivers can learn how to solve common problems from one another and reduce the feeling

Table 8-3   Recommendations for Mental Health Care

Condition of Caregiver	Recommended Type of Care	What It Provides	Where to Find
Fairly stable	Support group	Sharing how to solve common problems from one another Reduces the feeling that one is the only person facing such problems	Office on Aging, Alzheimer Association
Mental health problems Poor relationship with patient	Personal mental health care provider	Individual counseling	Social workers, psychiatrists, psychologists

that they are the only ones who face such problems. The caregiver who has significant personal mental health problems, however, such as a history of a poor relationship with the patient, may do better with his or her own mental health care provider than a generic support group. Support groups are not a panacea and must be recommended thoughtfully. For example, groups composed of sons and daughters of dementia patients may not be as helpful for spouses. See Table 8-3 for a summary of recommendations for mental health care.

Planning for the Family Too

It is evident that care for the family is as important as care for the patient and must always be included in any plan of care. The guidelines included in the Appendix can be copied and provided to caregivers and their extended families to reinforce these principles.

Chapter 9
PHARMACOLOGIC TREATMENT

Cynthia D. Steele

Key Points

- Two drug classes used to treat the symptoms of dementia
- When the use of pharmacologic treatments is appropriate
- The risks and advantages of using antipsychotic drugs with dementia patients
- The risks and advantages of using antidepressant drugs with dementia patients

Because there is no pharmaceutical cure for dementia, prescribers often focus on improving or stabilizing the dysfunction caused by dementia. The drugs that are available may have a limited effect lasting from 6 to 12 months. Pharmaceutical treatment is also available for the neuropsychiatric and behavioral symptoms of dementia. As a rule, nonpharmacologic and behavioral approaches to treatment are recommended before turning to treatment with pharmacologic agents.

It is important that the nurse has a sound understanding of the drugs that are commonly prescribed for persons with dementia, as this can greatly improve patient care. With this knowledge the attentive nurse can:

- Be watchful for potential side effects.
- Note the drug's effectiveness for a particular individual.
- Ensure titration and dosage are properly administered.

This chapter is more scientific than others in this book due to the nature of the content.

TYPES OF DRUGS FOR TREATMENT OF ALZHEIMER DISEASE

The United States Food and Drug Administration (FDA) has approved two types of medications for the treatment of Alzheimer disease: (1) cholinesterase inhibitors and (2) NMDA antagonists, which may temporarily improve or stabilize cognitive, functional, and behavioral symptoms of individuals with dementia.

Both classes of medication work at the synaptic neurotransmitter level only, and do not have any impact on the development of beta amyloid plaques and neurofibrillary tangles, which are found in the brains of patients with Alzheimer disease. These medications affect the activity of two different neurotransmitters, which are responsible for carrying messages between the nerve cells (neurons) of the brain.

Cholinesterase Inhibitors

Medications that increase the available levels of the neurotransmitter acetylcholine have been demonstrated to improve or stabilize memory and other cognitive symptoms such as language, judgment, functional abilities, planning, and other thought processes in individuals with dementia. Cholinesterase inhibitors have been best studied in patients with Alzheimer disease; however, there are limited data to suggest that they may be beneficial in the treatment of other dementia syndromes, such as Lewy body dementia, vascular dementia, and Parkinson disease.

How Cholinesterase Inhibitors Work

- Cholinesterase inhibitors reduce the naturally occurring breakdown of acetylcholine, a chemical messenger that affects learning and memory.
- This ultimately results in increased levels of acetylcholine that are available to help with communication among the nerve cells in the brain.

Available Drugs

Currently three drugs in this class are commonly used for the treatment of mild to moderate Alzheimer disease:

- Donepezil (Aricept), which recently obtained an indication from the FDA for the treatment of severe AD as well
- Rivastigmine (Exelon)
- Galantamine (Razadyne formerly known as Reminyl)

A third drug, tacrine (Cognex), the first cholinesterase inhibitor to come into the market in 1993, remains available but is rarely prescribed presently because donepezil, rivastigmine, and galantamine have more favorable side effect profiles and do not require frequent blood tests to monitor for possible liver toxicity.

Comparing Cholinesterase Inhibitors

Donepezil, rivastigmine, and galantamine are similar in terms of their treatment efficacy, so the choice of agent depends on prescriber preference, side effect profile, dosing frequency, and titration recommendations, which are described in Table 9-1. Both rivastigmine and galantamine were associated with a greater risk of trial dropout than placebo, especially at higher dosing levels.

Effectiveness of Cholinesterase Inhibitors

Individuals in the early and middle stages of Alzheimer disease (Mini-Mental State Exam score > 10) who do not suffer from co-morbid medical disorders or behavioral disorders have a 50% chance of modest short-term improvement, or more commonly stabilization, in memory and/or function on these medications that will last for approximately 6 to 12 months. There are some experts who believe that a small percentage of individuals with Alzheimer disease may benefit more in terms of symptom improvement and duration of action of these medications; however, more research needs to be done.

Side Effects of Cholinesterase Inhibitors

- The most common side effects of the cholinesterase inhibitors are gastrointestinal, and include nausea, diarrhea, vomiting, anorexia, and/or weight loss.

Table 9-1 Commonly Prescribed Cholinesterase Inhibitors

Agent	Dose Range	Administration	Titration	Minimum Effective Oral Dose
Donepezil (Aricept)	5–10 mg qd	Tablet; take with or without food	Start at 5 mg QHS for 4–6 weeks, and then increase to 10 mg QHS as tolerated	5 mg qd
Rivastigmine (Exelon)	1.5–6 mg bid	Tablet, oral solution, and patch; oral forms should be taken with food; patch should be applied to clean, dry intact skin and rotate the application site	For oral administration, start at 1.5 mg bid for 2–4 weeks, then if tolerated increase to 3 mg bid for 2–4 weeks, then 4.5 mg bid for 2–4 weeks, then 6 mg bid. Should be taken with a full meal. Initially apply one 4.6 mg/24 hr patch; if tolerated, may increase to 9.5 mg/24 hr patch after 4–6 weeks at previous dose.	3 mg bid in oral form 4.6 mg/24 hr in patch form
Galantamine (Razadyne formerly known as Reminyl)	4–12 mg bid	Tablet or oral solution; take with food. Also available in an extended-release form (Razadyne ER) which can be taken once a day	Start at 4 mg bid for 4–6 weeks, then increase to 8 mg bid for 4–6 weeks, then 12 mg bid as tolerated	8 mg bid, or 16 mg qd in ER form

- Rarely, cholinesterase inhibitors can cause bradycardia, syncope, and exacerbations of asthma symptoms.
- A small number of patients report a new onset of vivid dreams or nightmares while taking these medications. This can usually be managed by a slight reduction in the dose, and/or by avoiding bedtime administration of the medication.

Assessing Clinical Response

When a patient is started on a cholinesterase inhibitor, his or her clinical response should be assessed carefully by at least one and preferably several of the methods listed below.

1. A standardized measure of cognition, such as the Mini-Mental State Examination
2. A measure of overall functioning, such as an ADL scale
3. A clinician assessment of memory during the mental status exam
4. The historical opinion of one or more caregivers who know the patient well

Titration

Assuming that the patient tolerates the medication from a side effect standpoint, titration of the cholinesterase inhibitor should be completed no faster than is recommended in the package insert to the maximum daily dose. If there is no clear improvement or benefit from the medication after a period of 6 months at the maximum tolerated dose, then a trial off of the medication is indicated.

Comparison of Pharmacologic Properties

- The three commonly used cholinesterase inhibitors share a similar mechanism of action, but differ in other pharmacologic properties.
- There is limited evidence that patients who do not achieve clinical benefit from one of the cholinesterase inhibitors may still tolerate and experience benefit for a trial of an alternate cholinesterase inhibitor, although this has not become a routine part of care for patients with Alzheimer disease.

- If there have been no safety or tolerability issues with the initial cholinesterase inhibitor, the patient can be switched from one cholinesterase inhibitor to another without a washout period.
- If the patient *has* experienced problems with safety or tolerability with the initial medication, then a washout period of 7 to 14 days should be used to allow for resolution of any adverse side effects.
- There is no evidence to suggest that taking two different cholinesterase inhibitors at the same time would be more helpful than taking one alone. Combining cholinesterase inhibitors would likely result in a significantly greater frequency of side effects.

Additional Considerations

Many medications have anticholinergic side effects, which can decrease the efficacy of cholinesterase inhibitors. These include medications for overactive bladder, antihistamines, tricyclic antidepressants, and antipsychotics. It is not uncommon for patients with dementia to be taking cholinesterase inhibitors along with anticholinergic drugs. The practice of prescribing anticholinergic medications is generally discouraged in patients with dementia because of lessening the efficacy of cholinesterase inhibitors. Even when given independently of a cholinesterase inhibitor, they can cause delirium and other central nervous system side effects.

N-Methyl-D-Aspartate Antagonists

A second class of drugs, N-methyl-D-Aspartate (NMDA) antagonists, can be used alone or taken in combination with one of the cholinesterase inhibitors for a possible synergistic effect. Memantine (Namenda) is an NMDA receptor antagonist approved by the FDA for treatment of moderate to severe Alzheimer disease.

How Memantine Works

In Alzheimer disease, abnormal amounts of the neurotransmitter glutamate are released, causing damage to neurons. Glutamate is prevalent in regions of the brain associated with memory. Memantine works by blocking the activity caused by abnormally high or low levels of glutamate in the brain. Like the cholinesterase inhibitors, improvement in cognitive and functional symptoms is modest at best, and a decline in cognitive functioning seems to begin for most individuals after about 6 months.

Side Effects and Dosage

Potential side effects include headache, dizziness, constipation, and confusion. The typical starting dose of memantine is 5 mg qd and it is slowly increased by 5 mg each week or longer as tolerated until a dose of 10 mg bid is reached. It can be taken with or without food. Memantine should not be given to patients with severe renal disease, and to those who are also taking amantadine (Symmetrel) or dextromethorphan, because of their pharmacokinetic similarities.

Use of Other Agents for Treatment of Dementia

Patients, family members, or caregivers may ask about other potential medications or supplements that they believe may be helpful in treating the cognitive and functional decline in Alzheimer disease.

- **Vitamin E.** A single multicenter randomized trial indicated that 2000 IU of vitamin E a day may help to delay nursing home placement and functional disability among individuals with Alzheimer disease compared to placebo or selegiline. Recent research findings, however, indicate that individuals who take more than 400 IU of vitamin E a day were associated with a significant increase in mortality. Based on current evidence, patients who take vitamin E should be counseled not to take more than 400 IU qd and should avoid taking vitamin E if they are already taking antiplatelet or anticoagulant medications because of the possible risk of bleeding.

- **Anti-inflammatory medications.** Nonsteroidal antiinflammatory medications and prednisone have not demonstrated any benefit in the treatment of patients with Alzheimer disease.

• **Estrogen.** Hormone replacement therapy with estrogen has not demonstrated any benefit in the prevention or treatment of patients with Alzheimer disease, and may in fact result in more cognitive deficits than in those individuals taking a placebo.

PHARMACOLOGIC TREATMENT OF NEUROPSYCHIATRIC AND BEHAVIORAL SYMPTOMS

When Pharmacologic Treatment Should Be Used

A majority of individuals with dementia will develop one or more other neuropsychiatric or behavioral symptoms at some point during the course of their illness. Appropriate interventions for these common complicating symptoms—such as depression, mania, delusions, hallucinations, sleep disturbance, apathy, anxiety, and aggressive behaviors—are critical for the quality of life of patients and their caregivers. Due to the risks inherent with any pharmacologic intervention, nonpharmacologic interventions such as adaptations of the environment and adjustments in caregiver interactions should always be tried first. These important nonpharmacologic approaches are well described throughout this pocket guide.

In addition, before consideration is given to pharmacologic management of a dementia-related neuropsychiatric symptom, the astute nurse should consider whether the patient is experiencing an acute change in mental status and behavior due to a medical problem. See Box 9-1 for examples.

If nonpharmacologic approaches have been applied consistently and have failed to adequately reduce the frequency and severity of dangerous behavioral symptoms that might cause harm to the patient or others, then the introduction of a medication may be appropriate. It will still need to be carefully and routinely monitored over time, however.

The risk and potential benefits of any medication must be discussed with the patient (when appropriate) and/or the

Box 9-1 **Medical Problems Can Cause Change in Mental Status**

Potential causes of a patient's mental status should be ruled out and active medical problems should be addressed before consideration is given to specific pharmacologic management of neuropsychiatric symptoms of dementia.

Example: A patient with hypoxia from an acute exacerbation of chronic obstructive pulmonary disease may experience delirium with hallucinations and psychomotor agitation in the context of a delirium. Alternatively, the patient might also be experiencing changes in thought process or mood from a medication side effect.

Example: A patient who was recently started on levodopa for treatment of the motor symptoms of Parkinson disease may develop hallucinations or delusions.

Example: Depressed or labile mood may be seen in patients requiring anti-inflammatory treatment with prednisone.

patient's family/decision-maker. It is important for the nurse to be aware that no medications are specifically approved by the FDA to treat the neuropsychiatric and behavioral symptoms of individuals with dementia. The minimum amount of a medication should be used for the shortest time possible. The use of multiple medications to treat neuropsychiatric symptoms is more likely to result in negative side effects than the use of a single agent.

Overview of Neuropsychiatric Symptoms

Neuropsychiatric symptoms associated with dementia include delusions, hallucinations, agitation, verbal agitation, physical aggression, and resistance to care. This causes significant distress for individuals with dementia and their caregivers. Past research has demonstrated that 50% of individuals with dementia due to Alzheimer disease develop delusions and/or hallucinations over a 3-year period. Neuropsychiatric symptoms have also been associated with morbidity, mortality, and a higher cost of care for individuals with dementia. The most common antipsychotic medications, recommended laboratory monitoring, and potential side effects are outlined in Table 9-2.

Use of Antipsychotic Medications in Dementia

Historically, antipsychotic medications were widely used to attempt to treat the neuropsychiatric and problematic behaviors often associated with dementia. Conventional antipsychotics, such as haloperidol, have been available for over 50 years; however, in the past decade newer atypical antipsychotics became commonly used in clinical settings because it was thought that they resulted in fewer adverse reactions than the conventional agents.

Side Effects of Antipsychotic Drugs

Possible side effects of conventional and atypical antipsychotics include:

- Extra-pyramidal symptoms (EPS), such as dyskinesias (involuntary motor movements), parkinsonism (tremors, rigidity, shuffling gait), akathisia (internal sense of motor restlessness), and dystonia (spastic contractions of muscle groups)
- Anticholinergic symptoms, such as dry mouth, blurry vision, constipation, confusion, and urinary retention
- Sedation
- Orthostatic hypotension
- Weight gain

Neuroleptic malignant syndrome
While infrequent, there are some side effects of antipsychotic medications that are potentially fatal if not recognized and treated promptly. Neuroleptic malignant syndrome (NMS) is a life-threatening neurologic disorder that is almost exclusively caused by antipsychotic medications. The patient will typically present with muscle rigidity, fever, significant changes in blood pressure and heart rate, and an acute change in mental status.

Table 9-2 Common Antipsychotic Medications

Agent	Class	Lab Monitoring	EPS	Anticholinergic Side Effects	Sedation	Hypotension	Weight Gain
Aripiprazole (Abilify)	Atypical	Glucose if symptomatic	±	+	+	+	±
Clozapine (Clozaril)	Atypical	Weekly CBC, glucose, HgbA1C	±	++	+++	+++	+++
Haloperidol (Haldol)	High potency	Glucose if symptomatic	+++	++	++	++	+
Olanzapine (Zyprexa)	Atypical	Glucose, HgbA1C	±	+	++	+	+++
Quetiapine (Seroquel)	Atypical	Glucose if symptomatic	±	+	+	++	++
Risperidone (Risperdal)	Atypical	Glucose if symptomatic	++	++	+	++	++
Ziprasidone (Geodon)	Atypical	Glucose if symptomatic	±	+	+	+	±

±, minimal; +, mild; ++, moderate; +++, severe.

EPS, extra-pyradimal symptoms.

An elevation in the creatine phosphokinase (CPK) will help to confirm the diagnosis. The treatment of NMS is generally supportive in nature and discontinuation of the offending medication. The disorder commonly develops within the first month of the initial treatment with an antipsychotic drug; however, it has been known to develop at any time during the course that the drug is being taken.

Agranulocytosis

This is an acute condition that involves a severe and dangerous reduction in the number of white blood cells. One of the atypical antipsychotics, Clozapine, which is perhaps best known as having the lowest likelihood of causing parkinsonian symptoms, requires weekly complete blood count monitoring due to the risk of agranulocytosis and other blood dyscrasias.

Concern developed when atypical antipsychotics were linked to higher risks of cerebrovascular events and metabolic syndromes among older adults with dementia. This led the FDA to issue a black box warning for atypical antipsychotics in 2005. The health warning states: "Elderly patients with dementia-related psychosis treated with atypical antipsychotic drugs are at an increased risk of death compared to placebo." Further investigation, including results from the Clinical Antipsychotic Trials of Intervention and Effectiveness-Alzheimer Disease (CATIE-AD) and meta-analyses of antipsychotic use with dementia patients, soon demonstrated that:

- There were no significant differences found among the atypical antipsychotics.
- The risk of death mostly from cardiovascular and cerebrovascular events was 1.6 to 1.7 times greater than with placebo.
- Other significant adverse events included heart failure and infections, such as pneumonia.
- Adverse events may offset advantages in the efficacy of atypical antipsychotic use for treatment of psychosis, agitation, or aggression in individuals with AD.

Although not as well studied, the conventional antipsychotics seem to carry a similar, if not greater, risk of death than the atypicals. Based on available evidence, there is no support for switching older adults with dementia from atypical to conventional antipsychotic therapy for the purpose of reducing risk of stroke and/or death.

While the use of antipsychotic medications needs to be carefully considered in older adults, their use is not contraindicated and may help some individuals with dementia who exhibit psychotic, agitated, and/or aggressive symptoms who do not respond to other forms of treatment. Before deciding to treat with an antipsychotic, medical documentation should describe the reasons for prescribing the drug and outline the risk and benefit ratio. If behavioral interventions and other pharmacologic options have failed, psychotic and/or behavioral symptoms are severe, and there is an identifiable risk of harm to the patient or others without treatment, antipsychotics can be considered.

When prescribing antipsychotic medications, it is recommended to:

1. Start at a low dose and gradually increase the dose if clinically indicated.
2. Evaluate the need for continuing the medication after 3 to 6 months.
3. Periodically assess the patient's cardiopulmonary, cerebrovascular, and metabolic status.
4. Engage the patient's family members in ongoing discussions of the risks and benefits of treatment with this medication class.

Use of Antidepressant Medication in Patients with Dementia

Depression is one of the most common neuropsychiatric complications of dementia, and often presents in an atypical pattern of symptoms. Patients with dementia, particularly Alzheimer disease, may not appear or acknowledge feelings of sadness. Instead, they are more likely to demonstrate anhedonia (lack of joy in usually pleasurable activities), irritability, anxiety, psychomotor agitation, and mood-congruent delusions. Tearful episodes and low self-attitude are much less common or prominent, and frank suicidality is very rare. Depression in the context of a dementia syndrome may also be associated with mental suffering, sleep disturbance, striking out, weight loss, and social withdrawal.

Overview of Antidepressant Drugs

Antidepressant medications work by impacting the levels of neurotransmitters, such as serotonin and norepinephrine, in the brain. Antidepressant medications do not show any therapeutic benefit during the first 2 to 3 weeks of treatment, and 12 to 16 weeks of treatment with an antidepressant medication at a therapeutic dose is often needed to reach remission of symptoms or to deem the drug a treatment failure for that individual. There are several classes of antidepressant medications:

- Tricyclic antidepressants
- Monoamine oxidase inhibitors (MAOIs)
- Selective serotonin reuptake inhibitors (SSRIs)
- Serotonin and norepinephrine reuptake inhibitors (SNRIs)
- Other antidepressants such as buproprion (Wellbutrin), mirtazipine (Remeron), and trazodone (Desyrl)

Tricyclic antidepressants

Tricyclic antidepressants, such as nortriptyline (Pamelor) and desipramine (Norpramin); and monoamine oxidase inhibitors, such as Parnate, Nardil, and Marplan; are effective pharmacologic treatment options for depression. Their use with individuals with dementia is more limited because of their side effect profile.

Some common side effects of tricyclic antidepressants include anticholinergic side effects such as dry mouth, blurry vision, urinary retention, constipation, and cardiovascular side effects, such as orthostatic hypotension and arrhythmias. Monoamine oxidase inhibitors commonly cause orthostatic hypotension, and can cause potentially life-threatening hypertensive crisis when given in combination with over-the-counter decongestants (pseudoephedrine) or tyramine-containing foods (red wine, smoked meats, chocolate, etc.).

Selective serotonin reuptake inhibitors

The selective serotonin reuptake inhibitors (SSRIs) are the most commonly prescribed antidepressants for individuals with

Table 9-3   Antidepressants Used with Older Adults with Dementia

Agent	Class	Lab Monitoring	Serotonergic Side Effects	Anticholinergic Side Effects	Sedation	BP
Fluoxetine (Prozac)	SSRI	None	+++	−	+	−
Paroxetine (Paxil)	SSRI	None	+++	+	++	−
Sertraline (Zoloft)	SSRI	None	+++	−	+	−
Citalopram (Celexa)	SSRI	None	+++	−	+	−
Escitalopram (Lexapro)	SSRI	None	+++	−	+	−
Venlafaxine (Effexor)	SNRI	None	++	++	+	←
Mirtazapine (Remeron)	SNRI	None	+	++	++	↑↓
Duloxetine (Cymbalta)	SNRI	None	++	++	++	←
Nortriptyline (Pamelor)	TCA	EKG NTP levels	+	+++	++	→
Trazodone (Desyrel)	Unique	None	++	++	+++	−
Bupropion (Wellbutrin)	Unique	None	+++	++	−	←

SSRI, selective serotonin reuptake inhibitor; TCA, tricyclic antidepressant; NTP, normal temperature and pressure.

Table 9-4 Comparison of Anticonvulsants/Mood Stabilizers

Agent	Class	Lab Monitoring	Gait Unsteadiness	Liver Irritation	Sedation	GI
Lithium carbonate	Unique	BUN, Creatinine, Li+ level	++	–	++	+++
Carbamazepine (Tegretol)	Anticonvulsant	CBC AST, ALT Tegretol level	++	++	+	++
Valproic acid (Depakote)	Anticonvulsant	CBC AST, ALT VPA level	++	++	++	++
Gabapentin (Neurontin)	Anticonvulsant	–	+	–	+++	+
Lamotrigine (Lamictal)	Anticonvulsant	–	+	+	++	++

dementia due to their treatment efficacy and more favorable side effect profile for older adults. The most common side effects of SSRIs include gastrointestinal symptoms (nausea, vomiting, diarrhea), serotonergic side effects (insomnia, anxiety, restlessness), sexual side effects, metabolic disturbances such as hyponatremia, and weight gain. Table 9-3 summarizes some of the most common antidepressants used with older adults with dementia and compares their side effect profiles.

While selective serotonin reuptake inhibitors (SSRIs) have been effective in treating depressive symptoms in older adults with dementia, only one study of citalopram showed effectiveness in treating agitated and aggressive behaviors in dementia.

Anticonvulsants and Mood Stabilizers

With the risks associated with antipsychotic medications, some clinicians have prescribed anticonvulsant/mood stabilizer medications to control agitation in patients with dementia. Research in this area has been limited. Sink and colleagues found that anticonvulsants used as mood stabilizing agents, such as divalproex and carbamazepine, show mixed results regarding their effectiveness in treating neuropsychiatric symptoms of dementia patients. Common anticonvulsant/mood stabilizers and their common side effects are outlined in Table 9-4.

BIBLIOGRAPHY

Aggarwal NT, Decarli C. Vascular dementia: Emerging trends. *Semin Neurol.* 2007;27:66-77.

Auriacombe S, Pere J, Loria-Kanza Y, Vellas B. Efficacy and safety of rivastigmine in patients with Alzheimer's disease who failed to benefit from treatment with donepezil. *Curr Med Res Opin.* 2002;18(3):129-138.

Bentué-Ferrer D, Tribut O, Polard E, Allain H. Clinically significant drug interactions with cholinesterase inhibitors: A guide for neurologists. *CNS Drugs.* 2003;17(13):947-963.

Boada-Rovira M, Brodaty H, Cras P, et al. Efficacy and safety of donepezil in patients with Alzheimer's disease: Results of a global, multinational, clinical experience study. *Drugs Aging*. 2004;21(1):43-53.

Emre M. Switching cholinesterase inhibitors in patients with Alzheimer's disease. *Int J Clin Pract Suppl*. 2002;127:64-72.

Feldman H, Gauthier S, Hecker J, et al. A 24 week randomized double blind study of donepezil in moderate to severe Alzheimer's disease. *Neurology*. 2001;57(4):613-620.

Feldman H, Gauthier S, Hecker J, et al. Efficacy of donepezil on maintenance of activities of daily living in patients with moderate to severe Alzheimer's disease and the effect on caregiver burden. *J Am Geriatr Soc*. 2003;51(6):737-744.

Folstein MF, Folstein SE, McHugh PR. Mini-mental state: A practical method for grading the cognitive state of patients for the clinician. *J Psychiatr Res*. 1975;12(3):189-198.

Galik E, Rabins P, Lyketsos C. Dementia. In: Blumenfeld M, and Strain J, eds. *Psychosomatic Medicine*, New York: Lippincott; 2006.

Gauthier S, Emre M, Farlow MR, et al. Strategies for continued successful treatment of Alzheimer's disease: Switching cholinesterase inhibitors. *Curr Med Res Opin*. 2003;19(8):707-714.

Kales HC, Valenstein M, Kim HM, et al. Mortality risk in patients with dementia treated with antipsychotics versus other psychiatric medications. *Am J Psychiatry*. 2007;164(10):1568-1576.

Kaufer DI, Cummings JL, Christine D. Effect of tacrine on behavioral symptoms in Alzheimer's disease: An open label study. *J Geriatr Psychiatry Neurol*. 1996;9(1):1.

Miller ER, Pastor-Barriuso R, Dalal D, et al. Meta-analysis: High dosage of Vitamin E supplementation may increase all cause mortality. *Ann Intern Med*. 2005;142(1):37-W4.

Murman DL, Chen Q, Powell MC, et al. The incremental direct costs associated with behavioral symptoms in AD. *Neurology*. 2002;59(11):1721-1729.

Paulsen JS, Salmon DP, Thal LJ, et al. Incidence and risk factors for hallucinations and delusions in patients with probable AD. *Neurology*. 2000;54(10):1965-1971.

Rabins P, Lyketsos CG. Antipsychotic drugs in dementia: What should be made of the risks? *JAMA*. 2005;294(15): 1963-1965.

Reisberg B, Doody R, Stoffler A, et al. Memantine in moderate to severe Alzheimer's disease. *N Engl J Med.* 2003;348(14):1333-1341.

Ritchie CW., Ch B, Ames D. Meta-analysis of randomized trials of the efficacy and safety of donepezil, galantamine, and rivastigmine for the treatment of Alzheimer disease. *Am J Geriatr Psychiatry.* 2004;12(4):358-369.

Sano M, Ernesto C, Thomas RG, et al. A controlled trial of selegiline, alpha-tocopherol, or both as treatment for Alzheimer's disease. *N Engl J Med.* 1997;336(17):1216-1222.

Scarmeas N, Brandt J, Albert M, et al. Delusions and hallucinations are associated with worse outcome in Alzheimer disease. *Arch Neurol.* 2005;62(10):1601-1608.

Schneider LS, Dagerman KS, Insel P. Risk of death with atypical antipsychotic drug treatment for dementia: Meta-analysis of randomized placebo-controlled trials. *JAMA.* 2005;294(15):1934-1943.

Schneider LS, Dagerman KS, Insel P. Efficacy and adverse effects of atypical antipsychotics for dementia: Meta-analysis of randomized placebo controlled trials. *Am J Geriatr Psychiatry.* 2006; 14(3):191-210.

Seltzer B, Zolnouni P, Nunez M, et al. Efficacy of donepezil in early-stage Alzheimer disease: A randomized placebo-controlled trial. *Arch Neurol.* 2004;61(12):1852-1856.

Sink KM, Holden KF, Yaffe K. Pharmacological treatment of neuropsychiatric symptoms of dementia: A review of the evidence. *JAMA.* 2005;293(5):596-608

Tariot PN, Cummings JL, Katz IR, et al. A randomize, double-blind, placebo-controlled study of the efficacy and safety of donepezil in patients with Alzheimer's disease in the nursing home setting. *J Am Geriatr Soc.* 2001;49:1590-1599.

Winbland B, Kilander L, Eriksson S, et al. Donepezil in patients with severe Alzheimer's disease already receiving donepezil: A randomized controlled trial. *JAMA.* 2006;291:317-324.

Winbland B, Portis N. Memantine in severe dementia: Results of the M-Best Study (Benefit and efficacy in severely demented patients during treatment with memantine. *Int J Geriatr Psychiatry.* 1999;14:135-146.

Chapter 10

END-OF-LIFE CARE

Cynthia D. Steele

🔑 Key Points

- Most dementias are progressive and terminal.
- Decision-making about end-of-life care must begin early.
- Goals of end-of-life care are quality of life, dignity, and comfort.

The care of persons with dementia at the end of life (EOL) presents unique challenges to the persons themselves, their family members, and other caregivers. As most conditions causing dementia progress over many years, it may be difficult for families to realize that they are terminal in nature and advance planning is necessary. In addition, many families have never discussed issues of what the person wants and does not want in a terminal condition. The person with dementia may not be able to participate actively in many decisions due to cognitive impairment. However, those in mild to moderate stages who are dying of another condition may be able to be very actively involved in deciding their care preferences. Most persons with dementia die in nursing homes, and increasingly in assisted living facilities. Decisions about EOL care must be made explicitly clear to the care staff.

What are the characteristics of end of life in dementia? The clinical features of end-stage dementia have now been studied for a number of years. While different types of dementia have distinctive features, in the end stage the features are very similar. They include the following:

- Nonambulatory
- Vocabulary of 6 words or less
- Dysphasia (difficulty chewing and swallowing)
- Intercurrent infections such as pyelonephritis, pressure ulcers, and aspiration pneumonia
- Unable to dress or bathe
- Frequent urinary and fecal incontinence

The rate of progression to the end stage is different in different patients, so prediction of survival is inexact. In general, patients live 9 to 20 years until death. The most common cause of death is aspiration pneumonia and other complications of immobility, malnutrition, and dehydration. As described throughout this book, another way to describe the end stage is to return to the 4 A's of Alzheimer in the final progressive stage. These are summarized in Table 10-1.

Information on predictors of time of death has been identified in two major studies. The first, "The Predictors Study," followed a cohort of patients with dementia for 5 years and found that those who had psychosis (hallucinations and/or delusions) and extra-pyramidal symptoms (stiffness, tremors, shuffling gait) were more likely to die sooner than those who did not exhibit these symptoms. In another study, Volicer developed a

Table 10-1   Predictors of Death

Symptom	End-Stage Manifestations
Amnesia	Recent and remote memory severely impaired or nearly absent
Aphasia	Ability to say a few words, babbling, muteness
Apraxia	Unsteady gait or inability to walk at all, difficulty chewing and swallowing
Agnosia	Inability to recognize others or their environment

formula to predict life expectancy of 6 months or less in those patients who developed fever. Those who were older, had more severe dementia, and had palliative care in a hospital within 6 months predicted death within 6 months.

The following sections describe key concepts helpful in planning care and are adapted from the *Alzheimer Association Recommendations for End of Life Care in Assisted Living Residences and Nursing Homes*, 2007.

Active Dying

Active dying may include total body shutdown including heart and kidney failure, mottling or paleness of skin color, and cool extremities. The person may be unresponsive even though the eyes may be open, or he or she may be comatose and unarousable. A person in this situation has days or weeks to live.

Advance Directives

Advance directives are legal documents that describe a person's wishes for health care. While the documents differ state to state, there are two main types. The first is a Living Will. This documents your end-of-life care wishes in case you are no longer able to speak for yourself. There are many limitations with a living will. It cannot anticipate every decision that may arise. The common decisions such as resuscitation are sometimes easier to make than one to take you to the hospital for diagnostic tests. The second type of document is one that identifies a person who will make decisions for you when you can no longer do so. This document is a Durable Power of Attorney for Health Care, and allows this person only to make health care decisions and not financial ones.

While both types of documents are important in guiding care, the designation of a Durable Power of Attorney for Health Care allows for decisions to be made that were not addressed in the Living Will. The Durable Power of Attorney for Health

Care should ideally be given to someone chosen by the person himself or herself. It should be someone who knows the person well and can make decisions that are consistent with what that person would want or not want. In addition, a backup person should be designated if the first is not available.

While these are legal documents they do not have to be drawn up by a lawyer. A popular method of documenting a Durable Power of Attorney for Health Care and Living Will is called "the five wishes." It is simple and easy to complete. It can be obtained by contacting 1-888-5-wishes. It is legal in 36 states and the District of Columbia. The five wishes are listed below:

- The person I want to make care decisions for me when I can't
- The kind of medical care I want or don't want
- How comfortable I want to be
- How I want people to treat me
- What I want my loved ones to know

Hospice Care

Hospice care is palliative care for persons who are terminally ill with an expected survival of 6 months or less. This is prescribed by a physician and paid for by Medicare and Medicaid. This type of care can be given at home, in a nursing home, and in some assisted living facilities. Hospice services have been increasingly used for those with dementia in recent years since the broadening of terminal diagnoses to include dementia has been established.

Palliative Care

Palliative care focuses on alleviating physical, emotional, and spiritual suffering. It does not focus on curing a disease. Spiritual care assists persons and their loved ones to find meaning at the end of life.

WHEN TO START THE DISCUSSION ABOUT EOL CARE

The discussion between the clinical team, the person who is demented, and the family should begin at the time of diagnosis. This allows the person who is ill to participate to the degree that he or she is able. It also avoids the need to make decisions in a crisis situation. In many instances this discussion does not start until the individual is admitted to a care facility, which is not the ideal time.

Additionally, the family must be educated that when the patient is in the end stage he or she will not be abandoned but the goals and processes of care will be shifted.

GOALS OF CARE AT THE END OF LIFE

While earlier in the illness the focus of care is active participation in activities and maximizing physical health, EOL care shifts to quality of life, dignity, and comfort. This is achieved when the care is consistent with previous wishes, DPOA (Durable Power of Attorney) input, and the cultural and religious values of the person.

BENEFITS AND BURDENS OF MEDICAL INTERVENTIONS AT EOL

Cardiopulmonary Resuscitation

The cardiopulmonary resuscitation (CPR) outcomes for those in end-stage dementia are extremely poor. In fact, in less than 2% of cases that are witnessed is the outcome successful, and few of these individuals survive the subsequent hospital stay. Thus do not resuscitate (DNR) orders must be clearly documented in the person's medical record and known to the caregivers.

Tube Feeding

There is little evidence that artificial feeding via PEG tubes is beneficial to those in end-stage dementia. Weight loss is often inevitable whether a tube is inserted or not. Additionally, the use of those tubes does not decrease aspiration of food and fluid into the lungs. Complications from tubes are common and include dislodging, blocking, and infection. Such complications can result in admission to emergency departments and hospitals, which can be very traumatic for end-stage patients. Additional detriments of tube feeding include the need to restrain the patient to prevent him or her from pulling the tube out, lack of taste of food, lack of close contact with caregivers, diarrhea, nausea, and abdominal distension.

Treatment of Fever

This has been well studied by Volicer and associates and their findings reveal that efforts to diagnose the origin of the fever are successful only 30% of the time. He found that those with fever who were extensively evaluated and given antibiotics did not survive longer than those who were treated symptomatically with antipyretics and oxygen alone. Assuring light bed covers and the use of fans can also provide comfort.

Hospitalization

The transfer of end-stage patients to hospitals is often very detrimental to the patient. They must be transferred via ambulance, frequently need restraints, and are often treated by medical and nursing staff unfamiliar with such patients. Invasive medical testing often requires both restraints and sedation, increasing risk of further deconditioning and the development of additional hospital-acquired infections. IVs are often pulled out by patients as are Foley catheters.

Artificial Hydration

When patients can no longer swallow, dehydration follows. Terminal hydration often delivered via IV line has several disadvantages. It can result in fluid overload when other organs such as the heart and kidneys are failing. It is uncomfortable for the patient due to increased secretions and the possible need for suctioning and restraints. In contrast, terminal dehydration reduces secretions, limits coughing, and decreases urinary output, thus limiting the further complications of sepsis in decubiti.

GOOD CARE UNTIL THE END

Those with end-stage dementia must be given meticulous personal care. Some may call it modified intensive care. As stated earlier, the foci of care shifts to the following:

- Pain management
- Feeding
- Good skin care
- Bowel care
- Oral hygiene
- Maintaining dignity
- Spiritual support

Pain Management

There are many potential causes of pain/discomfort in end-stage dementia. These include contractures, just being immobile, and infections, which are most often urinary tract infections. While the recognition of pain/discomfort is challenging when the patient is unable to speak, there are some common indicators that can be recognized:

1. Noisy breathing
2. Negative vocalization, moaning, calling out

3. Sad facial expression
4. Frightened facial expression, furrowed brow
5. Guarding a body part when moved or touched
6. Tense body posture
7. Fidgeting

Since specific protocols are currently being developed for the treatment of pain in end-stage patients, several options can be tried. These include frequent repositioning and assuring that the patient does not have pain due to tight clothing or temperature in the room that is too hot or cold. It is essential that the staff determine that the patient does not have an infection such as a bladder or oral infection before pain medications are started. The previously described body audit is essential. There are many options for pain medication, from Tylenol to morphine. A staff that knows the patient well and can observe carefully can evaluate the effectiveness of both nonpharmacologic and pharmacologic interventions.

Feeding

Feeding is an emotionally difficult issue for families in the last stages of dementia. Common problems in this stage are listed below:

• Loss of appetite
• Inability to recognize food
• Refusal to open the mouth
• Sleeping through meals
• Inability to chew and swallow with the risk of choking
• Pocketing food in the mouth

Many measures have been suggested to help with these problems with feeding:

• Thickening liquids and foods as a bolus is easier for the body to recognize and begin the swallowing process.
• Giving lukewarm liquids, as the patients lack the ability to judge temperature and may be burned by hot liquids like coffee.

- Proper positioning of the patient with the head elevated at a 45-degree angle.
- Using a straw for those who can still suck.
- Sitting at eye level and feeding patients slowly, alternating between soft and liquids.
- For those who bite the spoon, substitute a small baby spoon that has a rubber coating on the end of the bowl of the spoon.
- Putting something the patient enjoys, such as ice cream, on the end of the spoon along with the food to get the process started.
- Stroking the throat from chin to neck.
- Feeding the patient in a quiet environment free from distractions.

Unfortunately, the inability to eat and drink is a feature of the end stage of dementia and families need to be educated that at some point attempts to feed their loved one are better stopped.

Skin Care

Vigilant attention to skin care is one of the most important aspects of excellence in EOL care. Documentation of reddened or open areas on the skin can help greatly in planning and evaluating interventions. In the elderly, the skin becomes thin and skin tears are common and in many cases unavoidable. An effort to avoid them includes padding the patient's arm extremities with towels, pillows, or sweatshirts when moving him or her. The extremes of moisture and dryness must be avoided. Soft mattresses and clothing can help irritation of skin, as can avoiding drying soaps. If the patient is in a wheelchair, pads that reduce sliding can help to keep the patient from moving out of proper alignment. The same is true for the use of wedge chair pads.

Skin shearing happens when the skin is pulled in the opposite direction of the patient's body. This commonly happens when a patient is pulled up in bed and the skin adheres to moist sheets. Drawsheets are useful at home and in nursing facilities, and assist in moving the patient and avoiding skin shearing.

Due to immobility, decubitus ulcers or bedsores are always a risk. Measures to avoid them include protecting bony prominences such as toes, heels, ankles, knees, buttocks, the sacrum, lower back shoulder blades, ears, breasts, and elbows. Such high-risk areas can be padded, but skin breakdown cannot always be avoided even with the most vigilant care. In addition, turning and repositioning the patient every 2 hours and using air mattresses that vary the pressure on the skin can also help.

Bowel and Bladder Care

Constipation is common in EOL patients. While it is recommended that a high-fiber diet be consumed along with adequate liquid (usually 2 liters/day), this is often not possible. Bowel movements and bowel sounds must be monitored daily and documented clearly. If no bowel movement occurs in 3 days, an oral mediation such as Milk of Magnesia is suggested. If that is unsuccessful, suppositories can be used. When they are needed, they are best given after breakfast. If such efforts fail and the patient routinely goes 4 days without a bowel movement, enemas may be used.

Urinary tract infections are also a risk with patients who are immobile and drink poorly. Direct care workers should be vigilant to a change in the color or odor of the urine and the frequency of voiding. As such infections are often painful, antibiotics are considered. Many new incontinence products have gel inserts and hold a large volume of urine. Nevertheless, patients should be checked frequently for wetness and changed as frequently as needed to avoid rashes and further infections. Wet or soiled incontinence products should be put in plastic bags and immediately removed from the room after changing to avoid the odor of urine or feces.

Oral Hygiene

Providing mouth care can be one of the most challenging care tasks at the end but one of the most important. Having a clean mouth and fresh breath is essential not only to health but also to dignity. Common care problems include dry mouth, cavities or broken teeth, and gum disease. Such problems are often the source of pain for patients but can also contribute to refusal to open the mouth for oral care.

Teeth should be brushed after the largest meal of the day. While giving mouth care, the oral cavity should be inspected and dried mucus and food particles should be removed with a moistened sponge-tipped applicator (commonly called a "too-thette"). If these are not available, a gauze wrapped tongue blade may be used as long as the gauze is securely taped to the blade to avoid aspiration. Dry mouth can be alleviated by artificial saliva, which is now available in small spray bottles. Thirst can be helped by the use of mouth swabs and ice chips if the patient can tolerate them.

Caregivers should not put their fingers between the patient's teeth. If the patient refuses to open his or her mouth, pressing on the cheeks and jaw can at times help. In many instances, it takes one person to do the care and another to hold the hands of the resistant patient.

Routine professional dental cleaning and care is ideal but often very difficult in the end stage of dementia. However, if a tooth is broken or infected, removal should be considered. The provision of good mouth care and oral hygiene can be very challenging but is an essential aspect of both health and dignity.

Maintaining Dignity

Care approaches that maintain dignity ensure a pleasant environment for the patient, staff, and friends and family. Such measures include the following:

- Keeping eyeglasses clean and on the patient
- Assuring that hearing aids are functional and kept in
- Grooming hair in the style that is customary for the patient
- Applying makeup if the patient is accustomed to it
- Keeping men clean shaven or with a tidy beard

It is also important to avoid hospital gowns and dress the person in his or her own clothes. This can be difficult when patients develop stiffness and contractures. Shirts that button in the front can be buttoned and cut up the back so they can be put on without turning the patient. The same can be done with dresses.

As always, the patient should be spoken to even if he or she seems unaware that another person is with him or her. Caregivers should continue to inform the patient of what they are doing before they begin. Gentle touch can be comforting and gains the attention of the patient before care is given. As reviewed earlier in this book, if two caregivers are required, one should do the care while the other talks to the patient. The decision of who will do the care and who will talk should be discussed before approaching the patient. Caregivers should never talk about the patient as if he or she was not there. Restraints should be avoided, as they most always increase discomfort and anxiety of the patient.

Seizures

Seizures at the end stage of dementia occur in approximately 10% of patients. If they result in possible injury to the patient, anticonvulsants can be considered. If the patient is in bed and the bedrails padded, in many cases such medications, which can result in excessive drowsiness, can be avoided. Families are often frightened by seizures and need education about the utility of keeping the patient safe and the possible use of medications.

Spirituality

The caregivers should know what spiritual and/or religious practices were important to the patient earlier in life. Singing hymns or playing familiar music can be a great comfort. As many learn basic prayers early in life, they can be read to the patient in the end. The custom of caring for the terminally ill differs by culture and religious belief, and as patient populations are getting more diverse, such customs must be respected.

HELPING FAMILIES

Families are best helped at the end through clear communication of the condition of the patient. It is common for visits with a mute and immobile patient to be awkward. Since it is very difficult to predict when the end is imminent, many families maintain a vigil for many days or hours at the bedside not knowing what to do. They should be instructed on giving comfort measures such as gentle stroking of the hands and arms, applying soothing lotions, and moistening the lips. One aspect of active dying is irregular breathing patterns such as Cheyne–Stokes breathing. This is evident when the patient takes a deep breath followed by shallower and shallower breaths and a period of apnea. If families are educated about this pattern they are less frightened by it.

Staff should allow families to visit as often as they feel they need to and should offer blankets or cots to stay at night if requested. Snacks and meals should be offered if possible. One way to bring closure and a sense of meaning to the patient's life is to encourage family members to talk about the patient and reminisce about his or her life before the illness.

When the end is near, it is not unusual for family strife to arise. This is the case when family members come together who have not been directly involved in the care of the patient. This is often called "the daughter from California syndrome." A typical scenario is for the uninvolved person to rush in and criticize the care that has been done by the primary caregiver. In such cases it is helpful for professional staff to have a meeting with the family members and explain the rationale for the care being given or withheld.

AFTER THE DEATH

Families are faced with several common issues upon the death of the patient. Even when loved ones are well educated, the death of the patient can be extremely upsetting. This acute grief can be surprising to caregivers who will often wonder why they were so upset when they knew it was coming. That illustrates the difference between the intellectual understanding of the illness and the emotional reaction to it. Such persons should be reassured that their feelings are normal for many.

Due to the long duration of dementia, some caregivers are relieved at the death of the patient and feel guilty. Those who converge for the funeral may be critical of that sense of relief. The end of the long saga of care giving results in the need for the caregiver to reorganize and fill his or her time. This process varies individually. Different family members will move through the grieving process in their own way and time.

The issue of whether the diagnosis of the type of the dementia should be confirmed by autopsy should be addressed early on, but often is not until the patient has died. Experienced professionals have good accuracy for the diagnosis during life. Since the clinical diagnosis is accurate in over 90% of cases, autopsy is not required. When the diagnosis has been unclear, autopsy findings can assist families and often provide reassurance that all possible treatments were offered. Autopsy findings also importantly contribute to knowledge through research. Again, knowledge of the religious practices of the patient and family will inform the caregivers if an autopsy would be acceptable to them or not. They should be told that if the brain is removed, an open-casket viewing can be done and there will be no visible signs of the procedure.

CONCLUSIONS

The care of the dementia patient in the end stage can be arduous for staff and family members alike. If they are prepared with the knowledge and skills described in this chapter, the process of care has a structure and roadmap. This minimizes anxiety and reassures everyone that they did all that was possible.

BIBLIOGRAPHY

The Alzheimer Association. *Dementia Care Practice Recommendations, Phase 3: End-of-Life Care*. The Alzheimer Association; Chicago, Illinois, 2007.

Carlson MC, Brandt J, Steele C, Baker A, Stern Y, Lyketsos CG. Predictor index of mortality in dementia patients. *J Gerontol A Biol Sci Med Sci*. September, 2001;56(9):M567-M570.

End of Life: Helping with Comfort and Care. Bethesda: National Institute on Aging, National Institutes of Health; January 2008.

Mitchell SL, Teno JM, Kelly DK, Schaffer ML, Jones RN, Prigerson HG, Volicer L. The clinical course of advanced dementia. *N Engl J Med*. October 15, 2009;361(16):1529-1538.

Rabins PV, Lyketsos G, Steele C. *Practical Dementia Care*. 2nd ed. Oxford: Oxford University Press; 2006.

Volicer L. Goals of care in advanced dementia: Quality of life, dignity and comfort. *J Nutr Health Aging*. November-December, 2007; 11(6):481.

FAMILY GUIDELINES

Cynthia D. Steele

FAMILY GUIDELINES SERIES # 1: WHAT IS DEMENTIA?

In the past, terms like "senility," "organic brain syndrome," or "late life confusion" were used to describe the elderly person who had difficulty thinking and remembering. The understanding of what is normal aging and what is abnormal aging has progressed so that new terms are used. The medical definition of dementia is the following:

A <u>global decline</u> in intellectual abilities of <u>sufficient severity</u> to <u>interfere</u> with occupational and or social functioning. This occurs in <u>clear consciousness.</u>

What does this mean?

- *Global decline* means that more than one aspect of thinking is affected. A person who only has memory problems or who only has difficulty in speaking would not be described as demented. Persons who are demented have memory impairment and difficulty in communicating, making decisions, and planning.

- *Sufficient severity* to impair functioning means that the problems the patient has are severe enough to produce problems in his or her daily life. Common problems include not remembering to pay bills; not being able to plan, shop, and prepare meals; and getting lost in familiar places.

- *Clear consciousness* means that the person is awake and alert. This is in contrast to a person who is drowsy and not able to pay attention or sustain attention due to an illness such as pneumonia and fever or who is impaired by medications, anesthesia, or alcohol.

What Causes Dementia?

Some conditions can mimic dementia and must be identified and treated. These include depression, intoxication from medications both prescription and over-the-counter herbs, thyroid disease, and anemia.

There are many causes of dementia. Some get worse over time and some do not. Causes include strokes, Parkinson disease, Huntington disease, and many others. Alzheimer disease (AD) is the most common cause. It can be diagnosed accurately and a variety of treatments are currently available.

FAMILY GUIDELINES SERIES # 2: ALZHEIMER DISEASE

Alzheimer disease (AD) is the most common cause of dementia in later life. AD begins gradually and gets worse over a period of years. The common symptoms of AD begin with the letter A and are known as the 4 A's of AD. Each of the symptoms causes difficulty in daily life.

- **Amnesia** (*Memory*). AD causes difficulty in registering new memories and recalling them. Common examples include the patient asking the same question over and over, and losing belongings. These problems occur because the part of the brain involved in registering new memories is damaged.
- **Aphasia** (*Language*). AD impacts on the ability of the patient to communicate with others and to understand what is being said to him or her. Many patients develop difficulty in finding words and their speech becomes vague and empty. Second, patients will have difficulty in understanding what is being said to them. Language problems are frustrating for both the patient and caregiver.

- **Apraxia** (*Doing things*). AD damages the parts of the brain that are involved in planning and directing the body to do things. Common examples are putting on clothing backwards and picking up food with the hands instead of using a knife and fork. Tasks must be simplified for the patient who has this symptom. Often, starting a task such as putting food on a fork and handing it to the patient can get a task started.

- **Agnosia** (*Recognizing the world*). Though patients with AD can see the world, brain disease causes difficulty in recognizing what they see. Common examples of this are the person who stands in front of the refrigerator looking at the milk but is unable to recognize it. Some patients who may be unable to recognize their caregiver become uncooperative or run away from them.

FAMILY GUIDELINES SERIES # 3: EATING

Many persons with Alzheimer disease will develop difficulty with eating and will lose weight. There are many causes of decreased eating including the patient not remembering if he or she has eaten or not, inability to ask for food due to language problems, inability to open complicated packages and to prepare meals, and inability to find or recognize food and drinks. Also, any source of pain such as dental pain can reduce eating and drinking. The following tips may help:

- Provide meals in a quiet and uncluttered place. TV and other noise can be too distracting for the person with AD.

- Serve one type of food at a time in small amounts. Too many choices can be overwhelming.

- Use simple place settings such as a contrasting plate and placemat and a single utensil.

- Provide meals on a routine schedule and have snacks and fluids readily visible for the person who needs to eat and drink more.

- Provide drinks every 2 hours instead of asking the person if he or she is thirsty.

- When patients can no longer cut up food, cut it in the kitchen before serving to preserve the person's dignity.

- If patients choke on thin liquids, add thickeners available at pharmacies. Maintain dental health by regular trips to the dentist or hygienist.
- If the patient eats very little, boost nutrition by adding calories to regular diet. Sometimes, putting something sweet on the tip of the spoon will encourage eating.
- Finger foods will make eating easier for persons who can no longer use utensils.

FAMILY GUIDELINES SERIES # 4: DRESSING

Getting patients with dementia dressed can be a challenge. The process of dressing can break down at many steps including inability to choose clothing, difficulty in putting it on correctly, wearing the same clothes over and over, and refusing to change clothes. As with other complicated tasks, one must determine where in the process the patient is having trouble and provide the help that is needed.

Suggestions

- Limit the choices: clear out a closet and place an acceptable outfit in clear view.
- Allow ample time: schedule appointments in late morning or in the afternoon. Rushing a patient can stall the process and upset everyone.
- Remove soiled clothing out of sight when the patient is bathing. Replace with clean clothing.
- Obtain clothing that is easy to put on and to take off. Jogging outfits, elastic-waist pants, shoes with Velcro straps, and clip-on neckties can allow maximum independence.
- Purchasing sets of similar clothing from catalogs can help if the patient insists on wearing the same thing over and over.
- Be prepared for opportunities to change. If the patient resists changing, keep spare underwear and clothing in the bathroom so that as the patient is sitting on the toilet and half undressed, clean clothing can quickly be put on.

- Be flexible: if arguments arise about changing clothes, drop the topic and try again later. Sometimes it is better to let the patient sleep in his or her clothes and attempt to change the next morning.

FAMILY GUIDELINES SERIES # 5: BATHING

Problems with bathing are very common in the care of those with dementia. Patients can become uncooperative with bathing for several reasons. They may have forgotten how to bathe, are frightened and cold, or don't recognize their caregiver. Many interpret attempts to bathe them as "someone trying to harm them."

Suggestions

- Build on past routines. If the person always took showers, he or she may not resist that as much as tub baths.
- Get organized: gather soap, towels, washcloths, and clean clothes ahead of time.
- Fill the tub ahead of time to decrease frightening noise.
- Plan the bath at the time the patient is rested and most cooperative.
- Give instructions one step at a time.
- Assure that the patient is warm by covering him or her with a large towel or flannel sheet and washing one body part at a time. Purchase a terrycloth robe to put on as soon as the bath is finished. That will begin the drying process and assure privacy and warmth.
- Give the patient the soap and washcloth so he or she can begin the process.
- A hand-held showerhead on a flexible cable can allow the caregiver to wash the patient easily.
- Obtain a shower or tub bench and install grab bars to avoid slipping. Put a towel on the bench to avoid slipping and to provide comfort.

FAMILY GUIDELINES SERIES # 6: GETTING TO THE BATHROOM

Losing control of bladder and bowels is not expected in dementia until the late stages. Earlier on, patients can have accidents for many reasons. With good planning, accidents can usually be avoided. Patients can become easily distracted and not realize they need to go until it is too late. They may forget where the bathroom is. Complicated clothing may take too long to undo. They may not recognize the toilet and may use other things like trashcans instead.

Suggestions

• Establish a routine: asking patients if they need to use the bathroom is insufficient to avoid accidents. One must take the person to the bathroom at least every two hours.

• Simplify clothing: eliminate complicated clothing such as pantyhose, belts, and zippers. Replace fasteners with Velcro or eliminate them by using elastic-waist pants.

• Limit fluids in the evening and avoid caffeine to reduce the risk of nighttime accidents.

• Plan ahead: locate family bathrooms in shopping malls and airports. Always take a change of clothes just in case.

• If accidents begin suddenly, take the patient to the doctor for a checkup. The patient may have an infection.

• When travelling, stop at least every two hours and take to the bathroom. Placing a sign on the door of the bathroom "Helping ill relative in the bathroom" can enhance privacy.

FAMILY GUIDELINES SERIES # 7: STRUCTURING ACTIVITIES

Alzheimer patients gradually lose the ability to plan their day. Gradually, things they did in the past such as cooking, yardwork, and participating in hobbies become too difficult and can become frustrating. As they lose a sense of time, they may get up in the night and try to go to work. A routine of activities during the day provides security to the patient and promotes rest and sleep at night. Without a routine, many patients follow their caregiver around all day.

Suggestions

- Try to get the patient up in the morning and in bed at the same times each day. Keeping the patient up and active during the day helps getting a good night's sleep.
- Write down an order to the day allowing ample time to complete tasks such as dressing and bathing. This will be helpful to other caregivers who provide help from time to time.
- Think of activities the person liked to do when he or she was well. Break them down into short achievable steps and give praise for completing each step.
- Doing the same thing over and over again is reassuring and not boring for many patients.
- Physical activities and time outside are useful. Even scheduling a walk in the yard or around a shopping mall can be enjoyable.
- Having a schedule also helps in asking for help from others. One can directly say "Bob goes for a walk at 11 A.M. every day, can you come over and take him?"
- If the patient becomes tired in the afternoons, allow him or her to sit and listen to music or look at magazines but avoid naps if possible.
- Planning an activity the patient especially enjoys after dinner will encourage the patient to stay up so he or she will sleep all night.

FAMILY GUIDELINES SERIES # 8: COMMUNICATION

Communication difficulties are common in dementia, and often frustrating for both the patient and caregiver. Examples of communication problems include:

- Finding words, "tip of the tongue" experience
- Losing one's train of thought
- Understanding what is being said

Suggestions

- Make sure you have the patient's attention before speaking.
- Speak slowly in a calm, low tone of voice.
- Use hand gestures to demonstrate requests ("sit here," patting the seat of the chair).
- Use simple, concrete words.
- Simplify the message into one or two parts.
- Give instructions one step at a time.
- Reassure rather than reason an explanation. "I'll wait for your return" provides much comfort to someone refusing to attend a day program.
- Respond to repeated questions with simple key words or phrases.
- Try to provide the word someone is struggling to say.
- Observe facial and body language to better understand what the patient is saying.
- Listen carefully for key words.
- When trying to communicate, eliminate distractions such as radio and TV.

FAMILY GUIDELINES SERIES # 9: MEDICATIONS

Taking medications properly is important. Memory loss and difficulty concentrating caused by dementia make taking medications correctly a challenge. Taking extra doses can be equally as harmful as forgetting doses. When patients have more than one doctor prescribing medicine, the chance of mistakes is even greater. Supervision of medications is necessary even early on in the disease process.

Suggestions

- Take inventory.
  - List all the medicines, including herbs, vitamins, and supplements; the doses; the frequency; and the doctor's name on one card. Gather and store all medications in one area.
  - Check through the house to find medicines (including kitchen cupboards and bathrobe pockets, dressers, purses, coats, bathroom cabinets).
  - Take the list of medications to every doctor's visit for review.
  - Throw out any expired medicines or those no longer used.
- Early in dementia, supervise medicine.
  - Use weekly pill box organizers.
  - Count the number of pills regularly to check for correct use.
  - Make a simple schedule for patients to follow.
- When mistakes are noticed
  - Remove all medicine from the patient's possession.
  - Keep medications stored in a secure place.
  - Give the pills immediately when they are to be taken; pills left out may get lost.
  - Make sure the patient swallows the pill.
- If a patient refuses medicine, ask for liquid alternatives or check if the pill can be crushed and added to a favorite food such as ice cream or pudding.
- Be careful using "over-the-counter" medicines. Ask your doctor before giving cold and cough medicine or sleep preparations.

FAMILY GUIDELINES SERIES # 10: HALLUCINATIONS

Some patients with Alzheimer disease or other dementia will develop hallucinations. These can be distressing symptoms for both the patients and their caregivers. When they occur, the doctor should be informed so that treatment can be discussed.

These are real experiences for the patient and can be frightening to them.

- Hallucinations are the experience of seeing things or hearing voices when nothing is there.
- Seeing things, animals, or people are the most common hallucinations.
- Hallucinations may occur as a result of another illness, an infection, medication side effects, or anesthesia.
- When patients hallucinate after surgery, they may be frightened and try to run away from the visions, creating safety risks.

Suggestions

- Look for signs of an illness or infection. Examples include sudden onset of incontinence (wetting accidents), a cough, drowsiness, or unsteady walking.
- Let your doctor know this has happened.
- Provide reassurance. For example, you might say: "I don't see those people but I'll keep you safe."
- Provide distraction. Moving the patient to another room or changing activity can sometimes distract him or her.
- Stay with patients when they are in the hospital if possible to avoid the use of restraints and sedation.

    In contrast to a hallucination, an illusion is a misinterpretation of something that is there. Examples include:

- Seeing a tall plant in a darkened room as a person.
- Thinking that a door slamming is a gunshot.

    One can minimize illusions by removing clutter and making sure lighting is adequate, closing drapes at night, and avoiding glare on tile floors.

FAMILY GUIDELINES SERIES # 11: DELUSIONS

Many patients with dementia develop delusions. Delusions are fixed false beliefs. Such beliefs are strongly held, and patients cannot be convinced otherwise. Delusions can result in aggression and put patients and their caregivers at risk of harm.

Common delusions in dementia include believing that:

- Someone is stealing from the patient.
- People are in the house who are not there.
- Caregivers are not who they say they are.
- The patient's food or medicines are poisoned.
- The patient's spouse is unfaithful.

Suggestions

- Avoid arguing or trying to reason with the patient.
- Provide reassurance that you will keep him or her safe.
- Try to find things the person says are stolen.
- Inform the doctor of the delusions.
- Try to distract the patient. For example, if he or she is looking for a deceased mother, say "I haven't seen her lately but let's get a snack and you can tell me about your mother."
- Make sure the patient is safe and cannot wander out.

FAMILY GUIDELINES SERIES # 12: DEPRESSION

Depression is a common complication of dementia and causes needless suffering to patients and their caregivers. Once thought of as a natural consequence of dementia, depression occurs in 20% to 40% of patients and can be effectively treated. No one can "will" away depression by "being stronger." Many patients won't complain of feeling sad or depressed. It is most important to understand that this is a chemical illness much like diabetes and is NOT a normal reaction to the knowledge of having a dementing illness.

Symptoms of depression in dementia include changes in:

- Mood—tearfulness, loss of pleasure
- Behavior—irritability, uncooperativeness
- Appetite—eating less, eating more

- Thoughts—low self-esteem, fearfulness, guilt
- Sleep—difficulty falling asleep, awakening earlier than usual
- Energy—loss of energy, apathy, withdrawal

Suggestions

- Have the patient evaluated. Report symptoms to the doctor.
- *Make sure the patient takes an antidepressant regularly if prescribed.*
- Encourage small, frequent snacks and meals to ensure adequate nutrition.
- Encourage patient to get out of bed and change clothes despite refusals.
- Assist with change of clothing to promote good hygiene.
- Offer reassurance and hope, since it may take time for medicine to be effective.

FAMILY GUIDELINES SERIES # 13: DRIVING

The issue of whether a patient with Alzheimer disease or other dementia should drive is important. The issue of independence makes driving a sensitive issue. Problems driving occur when something unusual happens such as a child running out in the street or there is construction and detours.

Problems in driving include:

- Getting lost
- Using poor judgment
- Driving in the middle of the road or on the wrong side
- Driving too fast or too slow
- Not obeying traffic signals

Suggestions

- If you feel uncomfortable riding with the patient, or if you would not allow a grandchild to ride with them, begin steps to stop them driving.

- Enlist the help of your doctor in getting the person to stop driving.
- Disable the car if necessary.
- Provide alternate methods of transportation.
- Relocate or sell the car.
- Obtain formal driving evaluation if necessary.

FAMILY GUIDELINES SERIES # 14: TASK BREAKDOWN

Task breakdown refers to simplifying the steps of activities in daily life. Task breakdown helps to overcome frustrating problems like:

- Difficulty in remembering the steps of a task
- Becoming easily distracted
- Having difficulty coordinating movements needed to complete a task

Suggestions

- Write down all the steps of a task.
- Observe the patient trying to complete a task, in order to identify parts that are difficult.
- Eliminate steps of a task that are frustrating for the patient.
- Give instructions one step at a time.
- Give praise for the completion of each step.
- Begin tasks for patients by getting them started, such as holding a shirt and putting an arm through the arm hole.
- Try putting your hand over the patient's and guiding it during tasks like holding a fork to eat or brushing teeth. This is called hand-over-hand guidance.
- Encourage patients to participate as much as they can without frustration, such as allowing a patient to stir food when he or she cannot follow a recipe.
- Re-evaluate task performance regularly. Most patients will have more difficulty over time and will need more help.

FAMILY GUIDELINES SERIES #15: TAKING INVENTORY

By the time dementia is recognized, the personal affairs of the patient are often in disarray. Common problems include misplacing checks, forgetting to pay bills, hiding money, and/or repeatedly withdrawing money from the bank. Patients may be reluctant to allow someone to help in these matters. The first step is to take inventory of the patient's obligations and assets.

Suggestions

Go through the house to find the following:
- All bills and obligations of the patient
- The checkbook
- Account numbers and location of all bank accounts
- Stock and bond certificates
- Social security and insurance cards
- Advance directives
- Last Will and Testament
- Discharge certificates from armed forces
- Pensions and other retirement benefits
- Insurance policies

Consider the need for a power of attorney or guardian to manage finances. For jewelry of sentimental or monetary value, consider costume jewelry as substitutes.

THE MENTAL STATUS EXAMINATION

Date: _____ Interviewer _____
Resident Name: _____ Rm# _____ Site of exam _____
Resident, age _____ male _____ female _____

"I would like to ask you some questions about your thoughts and feelings. Is that all right with you?"

1. *Level of consciousness*
   Hypervigilant?   Awake and alert?   Drowsy?   Stuporous?
   Comatose?   Fluctuating?   Stable?

2. *Appearance and behavior*
   A. Dress (appropriate to age? weather?)
   B. Grooming
      Neat?   Clean?   Clean shaven?   Make up?   Nails clean?
   C. Motor behavior
      (Motionless?   Fidgeting?   Tics?   Looks   Sad?   Crying?)
   _____
   _____

3. *Speech and language*
   A. Is speech spontaneous?
   B. Hesitation?
   C. Word finding difficulty?
   D. Rate of speech (normal, slow, fast and pressured)?
   E. Rhythm?
   F. Volume (normal, whisper, loud)?

Sample of
speech:_____

_____

4. Mood
(Patient's description of their mood)
"How have your spirits been lately?" or "How is your
mood?" or "Are you feeling happy? Sad?"

_____

_____

(Vital sense)
"Do you feel like your usual self? How is your energy?"

_____

_____

(Self attitude)
"How do you feel about yourself as a person?
Sometimes people feel they deserve to be punished, that
they are bad worthless people. Do you feel that way?"

_____

_____

(Feelings of guilt)
"Sometimes when people feel low, they feel guilty
about things. Do you ever feel like that?"

_____

_____

(Hopelessness)
"How does the future look to you?"

_____

_____

(Thoughts, plans of suicide)
"Do you enjoy life? Is life worth living? Do you ever
wish that you weren't alive anymore? Do you ever think of
ending your life? If yes, How have you thought you would
do away with yourself?"

_____

_____

5. *Delusions*
   "How are people treating you here?"_____

   "Do you worry that anyone is trying to harm you?"

   _____

"Are people taking your things?"

_____

"Is anyone poisoning your food or medicine?"

_____

   "Any other worries?"

   _____

   _____

6. *Hallucinations*
   "Does your mind ever play tricks on you? Do you see visions? Do you hear voices? If yes, whose voice, what do they say?"

   _____

   _____

7. *Obsessional thoughts, compulsive behaviors*
   "Do you have thoughts you can't get out of your head? Do you feel compelled to do things? Like checking the doorlocks?"

   _____

   _____

8. *Cognition*
Mini Mental score was _____ points. He/she missed:

_____

_____

SIRs score was _____

Index

Page numbers referencing figures are followed by an *f* ; page numbers referencing tables are followed by a *t*; and page numbers referring box are followed by a *b*.